Turning Illness Into Growth

Understanding the Modern Healer

by
Randall Leofsky

A Survival Guide for the 21st Century

SunShine Press Publications

SunShine Press Publications, Inc.
P. O. Box 333
Hygiene, CO 80533
Web: www.sunshinepress.com
Email: sunshinepress@sunshinepress.com

Cover design by Bob Schram

Publisher's Cataloging-in-Publication Data

Leofsky, Randall.
   Turning illness into growth : understanding the modern
   healer / Randall Leofsky
   p. cm.
   Includes bibliographical references
   Preassigned LCCN: 00-102255
   ISBN: 1-888604-11-5
   1. Alternative medicine. 2. Acupuncture. 3. Mind and body.
   4. Health. I. Title.

RZ401.B81 2000   615.851

Printed in the United States
5 4 3 2 1
Printed on recycled acid-free papers using soy ink

Dedication

This work is dedicated to the learners of the world. The thoughtful humble inidviduals who insist on creating their lives from their own information even though the rest of the world is telling them otherwise.

Publisher's Note

The contents presented in this book contain references and opinions on healing and medical matters. The material presented herein is an educational guide for health care providers and laypeople. It is not intended to replace the services of a health care provider or to act as a diagnostic tool. Any therapy undertaken for physical, mental, emotional or spiritual ailments should be properly supervised by an experienced health care provider. The publisher disclaims any responsibility arising from the use of information contained within this book. Responsibility for using or application of the material contained herein is solely at the reader's discretion and risks.

If you feel you or others have a medical or psychological problem, consult with a competent health care provider before pursuing any course of treatment.

Acknowledgments

A most special thanks to Anne Knapp for taking on the challenges presented by sharing a life with me during this work. Your tireless editing, questioning and joint explorations of the manuscript have been immensely valuable to me personally. It alone made the completion of this book possible. Your ability to bring clarity from confusion simply by rearranging a paragraph is an art and talent most of us can only marvel at.

I am deeply grateful to my many patients and students for all they have taught me. This is your book.

Thanks to my many teachers for sharing their wisdom and information. Especially J. Krishnamurti for sharing that which is beyond thought.

Contents

Preface

Increasing numbers of people realize that health and illness are more than biochemistry. The changes in people's health and lives as a result of energetic healing are exciting. In some cases the ease with which dramatic results can be obtained appear miraculous to the uninitiated as well as to the practitioners who use energetic medicine daily.

Energy, spirituality and healing are not intuitively obvious even though they affect us all. Familiarity with energetic healing reveals its logical basis that is fundamental to all aspects of life. Energetic phenomena have a basic common sense quality to them. Once on the trail of discovery, those seriously seeking this information soon realize there are unexpected treasures to be found. The principles that are involved in energetic healing and maintaining a healthful state also lead to spiritual fulfillment and inner peace.

As a teacher and practitioner of acupuncture and energetic healing, I'm frequently asked to explain these issues to my patients and students. While experiential classes are necessary to truly understand, there are always questions that benefit from an exploration that has been thoughtfully organized. This book is an exploration and guide for people seeking to understand the spiritual and energetic practices necessary for healing. These are the practices and principles used by the modern healer. In many cases they are practices from ancient healing arts that have evolved into a more workable and effective form.

Spiritual and energetic healing modalities are developing rapidly. An ever-increasing body of knowledge must be integrated and disseminated to the world at large. This information is bringing us to the threshold of a paradigm shift that will radically change how we approach illness and even how we think about ourselves and our bodies.

The book and questions within are organized to help with your personal and professional discovery and utilization. It is a book for the layperson, to assist in understanding alternative medicine and guide informed health care decisions. Alternative medicine practitioners will find new information on energetic modalities, including psychic healing, and their relationships to more traditional healing methods, including acupuncture. The thoughtful person will find much to ponder in the exploration of the mental processes that lead to illness.

How This Book Came to Be

The information in *Turning Illness Into Growth* is a result of personal clinical practice, the art of living, and personal insights. Much like an artist who has been influenced by the art or music of those that have come before, many have contributed to my understanding.

This book was written because I would get sick if I didn't. Not just depression but physically sick. I had aches in the joints, back, neck and head; even mysterious tooth aches and a general emotional malaise. Sometimes the discomfort was mild and at other times more serious. Some days my knees would ache so badly I could barely climb stairs. Once seated at the computer and writing, the discomfort would begin to go and the malaise was replaced with joy and enthusiasm.

At first the writing was just free association, expressing my pent up anger and frustration with a healthcare system that didn't make any sense. At the time, I didn't understand the connection between articulation and feeling good or procrastination and feeling bad. Sometimes writing stirred up an old wound and the issue's painful energy invaded the body. Resolving an issue could take weeks until the understanding was complete enough to write about it.

Eventually, writing became a pattern of pulling my hair for several hours over a topic. Afterward, my body felt light, aches subsided and I was rewarded with tremendous energy, lasting several days. But, if I didn't work on the book, the old ache or a new pain tormented me until I went back to it.

Sometimes insights churned around inside me, producing frustration and grumpiness. I didn't realize where the grumpiness was coming from. On occasion, as my energy stagnated, the grumpiness intensified, creating lethargy and anger. My only salvation was to continue writing. Organizing my thoughts has been a very personal process and I am finally able to share them with you.

Expressing our wisdom is not always simple or easy. It is often unwelcome information to those who resist new ways of being. Expression is fundamental to learning and the vitality that brings a healthful life. I wish you the best of luck as you begin the path of exploration and develop the wisdom that brings grace and joy in its expression.

Introduction

The Word is Not the Thing

It is important to keep in mind while reading this book that the words are merely pointers to the facts or phenomena that exist in nature. The words and concepts are my attempt to describe phenomena that have occurred in my clinical practice. The words I choose and the reader's interpretation undoubtedly will create some distortions. Therefore if it is to be of real value, the readers need to verify the phenomena described by seeing them in action within their own lives. That is to see the facts for themselves. Any concept the reader forms from the words needs to be accompanied with an insight or watched carefully for validity in action. In this way one's life becomes a laboratory for life science.

Who Are We? How Did We Get Here? How Does It All Work?

Throughout *Turning Illness Into Growth* we will visit these questions time and again. For it is through our exploration of these questions that we will come to understand that disease is really about a need for growth and change in our physical-spiritual being. The exploration won't always be nice and tidy. Life is not nice and tidy. It is vast and often mysterious. Consequently, the writing style within this book often reflects upon the vastness of the subject and the untidiness of mind. The book may not appear to have a logical order, as there is no logical order to exploring a sphere. Rather one must start at any given point and wander round till he has covered the whole thing. Of course in the end, the explorer must knit all the aspects explored together. This can be a painful task or joyous one depending on the nature of the mind undertaking it. If all is processed sufficiently, it will yield moments of glorious insight.

There will be much for the reader to ponder and meditate on. It has been said that some questions must sit on the brain for thousands of years before their true nature is revealed. The questions throughout this book are intended to be more than mere rhetoric. They are stepping off points for the reader to participate and integrate the material into her own life. To see the truth of the issue for herself.

At this point it would be helpful to understand a few fundamental concepts. There has been an attempt to organize this book, in general, around the concepts that are fundamental to understanding the wise use of the healing methodology and modalities at the end of the book. It is the premise of this book that for any sane approach to healing (medicine) it is essential that spirituality and clinical practice be united. This is not an alternative medicine or healing book any more than it is a spiritual, philosophical or religious book. Out of necessity they are all of these rolled into one. They are inseparable and that insight is the force behind *Turning Illness Into Growth*. It becomes a vast and unmanageable topic at times, if not endlessly broken down into pieces. When there are too many pieces the book becomes fragmentary and hard to integrate. *Turning Illness Into Growth* hopefully navigates that fine line. Every attempt has been made to keep statements concise and simple. The axiom "less is more" guided the process.

While every attempt was made to keep the presentation simple and straightforward it is not light reading to be pulled off the shelf and devoured like a bag of potato chips. Rather each chapter is like a coconut that needs to be cracked open and then chewed upon thoroughly. Truth wasn't created to be put into words, and if it was easy to understand, then where would the mystery be?

Section I - *Disease and the Divine Purpose* lays out the philosophical groundwork that is the foundation for the rest of the book. It is intended to be a basic approach to metaphysics.

Chapter 1 - *Rent Asunder—The Human Legacy* begins with getting an understanding of the consciousness we inherit when we find ourselves embodied. The original meaning of the term *rent asunder* actually means torn to pieces. When we take a body in this reality, our spiritual wholeness becomes fragmented by the dualistic consciousness that we inherit upon birth. We literally inherit the consciousness (the legacy) of the whole of humanity for the last 10,000 years. It is not your consciousness or my consciousness, it is just human consciousness. It is a mindset that sees itself as separate. From this initial fragmentation all kinds of corruption begin to sprout. The seedlings grow into disease of every imaginable variety.

In Chapter 2 - *Creating Illness For Growth* and Chapter 3 - *Disease as Signposts to Revelation* we investigate the purpose that illness affords us. We find the often asked question, "Why me?" can actually be answered. If we know why, then can we find the cure? Should we just fix whatever is broken with a magic bullet or potion? Maybe you will discover just what a magic bullet looks like? In Chapter 4 - *The Growth Period* and Chapter 5 - *Taking Responsibility For What We Create* we learn what it takes to heal, to change, why time may be necessary for this process, and why some illness may be a good thing. We also explore the questions: "If I am healing, why does it still hurt? Is this really good for me?" Once we have brought about healing/change, then we learn in Chapter 6 - *Seniority—The Art of Owning Your Own Space* a key factor in maintaining a state of *relative* ease. Relative is italicized here because in this chapter we find out that owning your space often has everything to do with your relatives. Obviously it is far better to correct the issues and energy than to suffer through an organ transplant. Chapter 7 - *The Banquet of Consequences* describes a few things that happen when we fail to be senior in our own space.

Section II - *Self-Healing—The Fast Track to Wellville* is where we get seriously into our stuff. It is time to look at what really motivates us. Once we understand where our desires come from we can just step out of the "rat race" altogether. We explore the many tools we have available to do just that. We examine the issues that make us sick and the many avenues available for self-healing.

The material in Section II is presented before Section III - *Facilitated Healing and Growth* for the reason it should also come first in our lives. Ultimately, all healing is self-healing. Nobody is going to fix you. Maybe a surgeon can replace your liver but the healing is still up to you. Self-healing is really a matter of discovering how the cosmos works and aligning yourself in harmony with it. This results in a state of inner peace and consequently good health. If we manage this on our own first, we will have little need for the facilitators and surgeons.

Chapter 9 - *Clairvoyance* is the fundamental bedrock of the self-healing process. Clairvoyance is not a way, a path or a method. It is not about religion, seances or crystal balls, but it can be. Clairvoyance is not about predicting the future. Clairvoyance is about insight, the ability to tell truth from a lie. It is about perceiving information through your sixth chakra. Rebirthing or meditation can spark clairvoyant insights and visions or it can be developed and used consciously on demand. It is not intuition. Intuition is a process of the fifth chakra. Healing cannot take place without insight—without seeing the truth. This chapter explores some of the many ways to awaken this ability, and use in an intelligent and responsible fashion.

Chapters 10-13 delve into the nature of the mind and thought. There will be no inner peace without this piece of the puzzle. We have inherited a consciousness that has run amuck, that has little understanding of its own arrogance—a consciousness that does not understand *right use* of its own intellectual processes. For us to experience good health we must understand the nature of thought and the ways of self centered consciousness. Once this is understood we move on in Chapters 14-16 and discover what it takes to align the energy with your new intellectual understanding so that real change can take place. We can't change the way we think, and create a fresh new page in our life if we don't clear the residue of the old ways out of the body. These old energies or *cosmic debris* will keep us locked into a feedback loop creating more havoc for ourselves. Once we have cleaned up our act we come to Chapter 17 - *Cooperation*. This is the unfolding of the blossom. The beauty of the human being is revealed. It's all about love!

Section III - *Facilitated Healing and Growth* oddly was the most difficult subject to write. We are talking about concrete tangible techniques instead of metaphysics, so it should be straightforward. The difficulty arises, as the outcome in any treatment often is more the result of how the healer's energy field interacts with the patient's field rather than from the technique used. One of my healers, a Rolfing instructor, in attempting to explain the difficulties in teaching bodywork or healing, summarizes the issue this way: "It is not what you do but rather who you are!"

Facilitated Healing and Growth is about exploring the different modalities and what they can do for you. Paramount to understanding the differences in these systems is that the practitioners of the modality often influence the results more that the method they use. Some bodyworkers can balance your energy system without realizing they are working with energy. They may have the ability as spirit to heal you with psychic energies unknowingly, perhaps better than some energy workers can. Likewise, some energy workers can relax your muscles and align your structure more effectively than a bodyworker. Nonetheless, different modalities have different purposes and this book explores those intended purposes. If some modalities don't appear in the book it is because the author chose the modalities he finds most useful.

Chapters 22 - 25 take a look at medical science and its role in industrialized medicine. Particularly, are the cause and effect relationships between aberrant biochemistry and illness truly the basis for disease? Then a brief look at the for profit medicine and managed care industry from the perspective of the Hippocratic oath "If you can't do the patient any good, then do no harm" and the biblical admonition "Forgive them father, for they know not what they do." In many cases, they know what they do and they do it anyway.

Chapter 26 - *Stick Me, Pound Me, Bake Me, Plug Me into the Wall Baby* explores the therapeutic benefits of acupuncture, bodywork, hydrotherapy, and colonics. What treatment is best for what ails you?

Chapter 27 - *Working with the Woo Woo* and Chapter 28 - *Psychic Healing* explore cutting edge healthcare. This will influence the medicine of the future even if it can't be packaged and sold for great profit. It works and it is easy to learn. Could it be a threat to the medical industrial complex? At some point the established medical community will likely usurp energetic medicine. Marketing firms will no doubt make claims that they can do the same thing with imitative machinery, only better because it is scientific. Can it be true?

Chapter 29 - *Healing with Color and Crystals* illuminates the possible consequences that can about from "tooling around" with too little information, and what to do about it.

Chapter 30 - *Reconnection* is about the idea that "all roads lead to Rome," and all paths lead back home to the Divine. Some journeys are just longer and more convoluted than others. We happen to be living in a time where we have the information available to us to take a direct route, even a shortcut.

Section I

Disease and the Divine Purpose

There are many lessons to be learned and scales to be balanced. The laws of the universe cannot be altered for one's convenience. Humanity must learn to accept everything that life offers as a learning experience. It is for this reason that spiritually immature people cannot be spoon-fed by someone else. The seeker must walk alone—with God.

—Peace Pilgrim

Chapter 1

A man identifies with a small problem that confronts him and he completely forgets the great aims with which he began his work. He identifies with one thought and forgets other thoughts; he is identified with one feeling, with one mood, and forgets his own wider thoughts, emotions and moods...When he can cease identifying with himself—and this will happen when he stops using the term 'I'—he will then remember his essence, his proper self.

—Gurdjieff

Rent Asunder
The Human Legacy

Upon birth, humans inherit a legacy of wholeness rent asunder by generations of fragmented thinking. We think of ourselves as separated into different races, religions, political ideologies, nationalities, sexual affinities and the list goes on and on. This fragmented worldview sets the stage inevitably for competition and battles of every sort. While one can learn and grow from this existence as one might from any existence with the pleasures and misfortunes of a body, the playing field is essentially a petty affair.

Spiritual beings at our level of experience are capable of so much more. This divisive and petty consciousness sets the stage for disease. The disease itself points the way to wholeness of body mind and spirit. Our body provides all the information we need.

Is this sense of physical separateness true? Are we similarly separate spiritually? Is it that we feel physically separate as individuals, but are united energetically as a whole, like cells in a body?

Why Me?

What are the origins of these beliefs of being so separate and so isolated? While the western medical model of how our bodies work has played a big part in the formation of who we think we are, it probably started much further back. Maybe the original sin was to buy into the notion that we are biologic organisms separate and distinct from the divine. It is perhaps the concept that we are only flesh and blood.

Yes, we are flesh and blood, but are we more of a biochemical machine than spiritual being? Most would probably answer yes; we are more biochemical than spirit. It is probably this concept more than any other factor that continues to keep us separate from the truth, of who we are. While our chakras are configured in a fashion to keep us in an earthbound consciousness, which keeps us cut off from our spiritual information, we are still spirit. Our biochemistry still responds to the higher enlivening vibrations of spirit energy. In human form we are caught between biochemical machinery and spirit, not wholly one or the other, but rather a synergistic blend.

Most of us grow up believing that illness is a random event. For example, we read statistics such as 1 in 4 people will contract cancer. Statistical analysis is a popular way of looking at illness. The implication is that illness is entirely impersonal, it is just a toss of the dice.

Biochemical and statistical explanations often feel patronizing, insulting, and inadequate. It's not that the biochemical explanation is wrong, it is more that the biochemical aberration is in itself an effect of a deeper cause.

Many of us who have had a serious illness have asked ourselves the question, "Why me?" Most of us seem to have an innate sense that there is a reason for it. Medical scientists have tried to answer the question by explaining the illness to the patient in terms of biochemical mechanisms. Often science has no explanation at all, but rather offers us the solace and stigma of the name of a disease or syndrome. In many cases these are merely arbitrary names given to collections of symptoms. Presumably this makes the patient feel as if the M.D. knows what the problem is and the patient must have come to the right place. Maybe it is really so the doctors themselves believe they know what they are doing. In the western medical model, medical doctors are lost without a diagnosis. If they don't have a name for a disease, they have no treatment.

There are closely defined and accepted protocols in western medicine, all based on the ability to give a name to the malady. If it is just a series of aches and pains and a little feeling out of sorts, catch-all terms such as depression are often given to patients, along with prescriptions to buy drugs. Then, they feel better because they are doing something for themselves. Probably more importantly, the doctors think they are doing something beneficial. If the patient is lucky, it will be a placebo. If unlucky, it may be something addictive like one of the modern mood enhancing drugs.

In the case of some diseases, such as emphysema in a long-term smoker and liver disease in an alcoholic, the connection is more obvious. The "why me" can be answered with because you smoked two packs of cigarettes a day or drank heavily for thirty years. There are also those who smoke heavily and don't get emphysema or lung cancer and live long lives. What is that about? One can still go deeper and ask why did one feel the need to smoke two packs a day. What is the energetic imbalance that set up the cravings? The role of abuse in most illnesses is usually not obvious or it is a result of many subtle energetic and emotional factors. These subtle factors in themselves could produce illness or create cravings and abusive behavior patterns that lead to disease.

The Body as Machine

The current paradigm for illness has been to look at the body as if it were a machine. Diagnose the part that is malfunctioning. Then treat it or replace it as if your heart was an oil pump on your car. Sometimes, why bother with replacing the part if it can still run or limp along without it? Just like a car can run without its air filter or a headlight, let the body run without tonsils or a gallbladder. The problem is similar to the car that can run without an air filter although the oil gets dirty faster and begins to wear out the piston rings. Oily black smoke begins to pour out the exhaust pipe. A body without its tonsils becomes more susceptible to infection. A body without a gallbladder will have difficulty digesting fatty foods.

Explaining illness in terms of biochemical mechanisms brings to mind the story about the lost keys:

There is a hip young fellow walking down a dimly lit street and comes upon this old man walking in circles under a street light muttering to himself. Wanting to be helpful he calls out, "Hey what's up dude?" The old man answers, "I'm looking for my keys." Eager to be helpful the young fellow starts scouring the pavement. After a couple of minutes he finds nothing. He asks the poor chap "So where exactly did you lose your keys?" The reply comes, "Over there, in the yard." The young fellow astonished, "If you lost the keys in the yard then why are you looking out here in the street?" The old man answers "There is more light out here."

Medical science is not comfortable in dealing with anything beyond a three-dimensional model plus the fourth dimension time, for a reality. The process of observing and testing precisely with its instruments becomes rather difficult. So there is a widespread denial that any subtle energetic (spiritual) forces exist. So focus the search where the light is, where the instruments can see. Focus then on biochemical mechanisms and, with a good public relations machine, people will forget all about the keys.

There is something that feels terribly unnatural about the western medical model. A model we inherited with our consciousness as we learned to speak. Even though we may not be scientists ourselves the basic principles of the scientific model of who we are is passed on subtly through the language we absorb at an early age. While science was wise to separate itself from the blind faith and historical miscreance of organized religions, it seems to have thrown the baby out with the bath water.

Medical science in its pursuit of the *magic bullet* seems to have turned a blind eye to many of its own who allow for spiritual energetic influences. Well-known researchers like Rupert Sheldrake, Harris Walker, Albert Szent-Gyoergyi and others acknowledge a force operating beyond the purely material. The time for marrying the scientific process with spirituality is overdue. Without this union our medicine, although possessing lots of technological wowie-zowie, is still primitive. It is high time we learn to work with the energy that is responsible for the biochemical aberrations.

Most of us, when ill, have a sense that there is a reason for the current malady. Somehow we feel we are not in the natural flow—we are not right with nature. Perhaps we did something wrong or unhealthy and now we are paying for it. Or perhaps, there is something we are supposed to learn from this experience. There are also those who believe that their illness is punishment for some dirty deed. This may sometimes be the case, but we will deal with that later.

If we know what was creating our illness, and why, it obviously follows that we might be able to change our behavior, thoughts, diet, environment and other factors to get right with nature again. Perhaps there is even something we can do ourselves to return to health, and not have to give our power away to the experts with all their drugs and invasive techniques.

For example, in the case study below, a woman's cancer started with repressed resentment. If in some type of therapy, she was able to access that stuck emotional energy and clear it from her energy body it would greatly free up the physical body to do its healing. If she was also consciously able to understand and deal with the emotions, it would help her better understand herself. She would learn how she creates events in her life as well as developing a better understanding of the world around her.

> *72-year-old female with liver and pancreatic cancer. Three children. Yoga teacher. With respect to oriental medicine we have wiry, taut pulses for many years preceding the cancerous stages of illness. Tight wiry pulses would indicate Liver stagnation, which would indicate the presence of anger. Anger that is not obvious, noticeable in the individual only by a sensitive, trained observer or a clairvoyant.*
>
> *From a biochemical perspective this person would be in a sympathetic fight or flight mode much of the time, this will affect a myriad of biochemical pathways summed up by the word "stress." When this person was looked at clairvoyantly during her fight with cancer, an unwanted fetus was seen. This fetus was not aborted. It was in fact her youngest son. She resented very strongly having another child, but would not let herself feel this emotion. Like most of us, she had perfect pictures about motherhood and having to love her son and would not let the resentment surface.*
>
> *This resentment, held in for many years, created much stagnancy in her Liver Qi. Over time this stagnancy progressed to Liver Yin deficiency and finally to cancer. A western scientist might*

*quickly point to many carcinogens in her diet or environment.
However, if she were healthy this would be quickly neutralized by the
body's defenses. This reading did not result in a miracle recovery and
she died two months later. It also was discovered in the reading that,
as spirit, she did not want to hang on to this body any longer, she was
ready for new things. While the body consciousness was clinging
valiantly to life, her spirit was pulling its energy out of the body.*

*When spirit and body are battling at cross-purposes, the body
doesn't win the battle for long. She also underwent chemotherapy,
and took many herbal remedies. She lived for nearly two years after
the cancer was discovered. This was a long period for a person with
liver cancer. Her body put up quite the fight, as she did many
healthful things such as the herbs and yoga to help fight off the
illness.*

Between Heaven and Earth

As human beings we exist between the heavens (subtle energy) and
earth (physical matter) not wholly one or the other. The qualities we
manifest as humans are a direct reflection of the spiritual energy that
enlivens the body. What is Spiritual Energy? It is the spark of the divine
that enlivens the body. It exists in the form of a subtle energy that is
distinct and unique unto itself. This energy field continues with or
without the body and contains a tremendous amount of information held
within it. This information is stored within this field much in the same
way as a computer stores information. We learn about that energy (who
we are) by the nature of its manifestation in our bodies. The nature of
that energy further reveals itself in what we create in our lives and the
manner in which we go about the process of creation. Disease is just
another aspect of what we manifest and each disease has a story to tell.

That story usually contains information as to the role of the disease
in our life purpose. Our clairvoyance is the instrument we use to read
that story. Developing the sensitivity and ability to do clairvoyant
readings can provide many answers to the "Why me?" in illness.
Clairvoyance is an ability we all have but have forgotten how to use. We
all get pictures that we can see with our third eye (sixth chakra) but we
have been taught not to trust them. Once again, another product of our
legacy of scientific materialism.

Becoming clairvoyant is a matter of learning to trust your pictures and developing the ability to interpret them in a neutral way. As with anything, clairvoyant reading comes easier to some people than others. Those who would use it to predict future time events have eroded the clairvoyant's credibility. We also inherit a legacy of superstition, witchcraft and misuse of our psychic skills. Predicting future-time events carries with it a heavy responsibility. When one reads future-time you are seeing only one of many possible futures. Solely by virtue of seeing a future-time scenario and describing it to the person involved will change the energy around the event. Changing the energy around the event will also change the likelihood of it coming to fruition. If it was the most probable future then it won't be any longer. At least from the probability of it now happening. By the same token when we look at a picture for the stuck energy around a disease it creates movement around the issue and changes the energy.

Those in the scientific community who would criticize medical intuitives have not developed their ability to see and test clairvoyance first hand. It is like saying you don't like tofu without ever having tasted any. This kind of prejudice and closed mindedness quickly separates the serious scientist from dilettante. The serious scientist's first and foremost concern is a curiosity for and about nature. The scientist who is a politician first, and a scientist second may wear a lab coat and have all the appropriate credentials. However, her deep interest is for position, power, prestige and material gain. This may sound like sour grapes but the inability of society to incorporate radical new paradigmatic shifts is always a political problem not an intellectual one. As a society it is our legacy to have suffered much from this short-sightedness.

Clairvoyance is quite simply the ability to see clearly or to tell truth from a lie, the ability to look from neutral. It is the power of discerning objects or information not present to the physical senses but regarded as having objective reality or actuality. The true beauty is in the ability to look at oneself with neutrality and facilitate one's own healing. The healing that comes with clairvoyance is primarily self-healing rather than using it to operate externally on others even though it has an important role there as well.

With an understanding of clairvoyant readings, oriental medicine, and western biochemistry we can now begin to get the Big Picture and have a better perspective from which to answer the question, "Why me?" This process leads to many discoveries along the way in addition to the medical one. We begin to see that our medical condition is not separate from our mental/emotional states. A model begins to emerge for how mental/ emotional states affect the physical body.

Illness essentially represents a breakdown in our ability to come to terms with an issue; it is stagnation in the growth process.

This growth is a process that begins with our individuation and matures with the realization of oneness. The qualities of our illness or health allow us to reflect on the nature of the energy that created it. In this way we have the potential to learn and grow. Either we express and exhibit our spiritual information or we deny it and get sick.

Chapter 2

I wipe away my tears of sorrow, finding it does not matter to thee whether I play a big or a small part, so long as I play it well.
—Unknown Origin

Creating Illness for Growth

Over many lifetimes we experience much growth and become proficient at the art of creation. Eventually we must take on limitations to our creativity so that we can be challenged to learn or study particular things. Where would the thrill be if we could manifest our every desire instantly? What would we learn? Illness is one of the many things we create as spirit to put us in a situation where we will have to develop specific abilities and talents. These are illnesses created for learning or growth.

There are many issues to be explored and understood as a result of our illnesses. Whether it is heightened sensitivity to energy derived from blindness, forced rest and relaxation from exhaustion, or an accident or debilitating illness that restricts one to a wheelchair, illness is no accident. It is not a random event. As spirit, we learn about the cosmos and ourselves by our ability to create. We create to see what works and what doesn't. This process of life is an exploration of the nature of existence. Spirit has no ethics about the type of creation—painful, joyous or otherwise. It is all learning, and that's a good thing!

There is a Japanese system of acupuncture based on the practitioner's ability to feel subtle energies. It is probably the finest system of acupuncture in the world. Blind practitioners developed the Toyohari Association's system of acupuncture. Their sensitivity to energy was heightened as a result of their blindness. This led them to radically different techniques such as stimulating Qi without inserting the needle. In this system, moving Qi achieves energetic balance while holding a

11

gold or silver needle over the point using a refined and specialized technique. Their illness allowed them to develop special skill that now will serve the world, as well as themselves.

There is a story from China that illustrates how our creations are not always what they seem to be. The story is about Mr. Li, an old man in rural China, and a beautiful and unusually intelligent horse, named Mystic.

All the villagers admired Mystic as Mr. Li rode him through the town. The villagers would say, "Mr. Li you are a very lucky man to have such a fine animal as Mystic." Mr. Li's response would be simply "maybe" as he rode on his way. This response puzzled the villagers but they smiled and went about their business.

Mr. Li rode and groomed Mystic every day, as he loved him very much. Then one night a windstorm blew a tree over, breaking the old wooden corral. Mystic wandered away in the night through the broken fence. Mr. Li was sad indeed. His neighbors responded to his sadness with their sympathy, commenting "tough luck" and "what an unfortunate occurrence" this was. Mr. Li again responded "maybe." As time passed, people forgot about Mystic.

Then one day, Mr. Li awoke to a commotion in the barnyard. Through bleary eyes he finds Mystic has returned, but not alone. Mystic led a pack of sixteen wild horses into the corral. Mr. Li was very grateful to have Mystic back and sold many of the new horses and profited handsomely. The villagers were all quite envious and commented on how lucky Mr. Li was. Mr. Li's response was still the familiar "maybe."

Mr. Li's son set out to train and break the remaining horses. One particularly spirited horse threw him off, breaking his leg. This was disastrous because harvest time was approaching and Mr. Li was feeble. On seeing this, the neighbors again commented on Mr. Li's bad luck. Still he had the same response, "maybe."

Soon afterwards, the conscription army came through town drafting every available young man for the army. Mr. Li's household was spared as his son had a broken leg and was unfit for duty. The villagers bemoaned the loss of their sons, and again commented on Mr. Li's luck. By now they all knew what his answer would be.

Trust

Mr. Li was on to the fact that there is no such thing as luck. You never really know in what form fortune may come, but it comes as a result of an ordered cosmos. This is the basis for trust. Trust is about remaining open to outcomes and being slow at coming to conclusions and judgement. It is our natural state of being, our background vibration when fear is absent.

Trust needs to be distinguished from faith, as they are not the same things. Faith is the state of being convinced that a *belief*, which may or may not be true, is the actual truth. It is easy to trust that there will be air for us to breathe if we walk outside. We don't think much about air, we just assume it will be there. This is trust; it is an absence of fear. If we create lots of fearful thoughts about ecological disaster, we may not be able to trust any longer. To be confident we would need to come up with a believable rationale that the disaster won't happen. This is faith; it's the damage control that comes after fear to make us feel safe.

Conclusion, judgement, and defensiveness (unlike trust) inevitably follow faith. Trust and stress are mutually exclusive. Stress is the by-product of anxiety and fear. Trust is necessary for optimum health and well-being. Faith is like a bandage on a wound or splint on a broken leg. With faith there will always be a stress (fear, anxiety, or uncertainty) buried somewhere in our psyche. As a result, what we create from trust will be vastly different from what we create with faith.

Most of us have noticed that animals can sense our fear of them. If we trust that the encounter with the big shaggy dog will be pleasant, it usually is. If we try to cover our fear of the animal with faith in a happy outcome, does it work? Do animals sense your energy, your body language or both? Can you tell when you are imbued with trust as opposed to faith? Our subtle energy system is the language we use for this communication. It is both the medium and the content.

The above example is a very simplified picture of how we affect the world (in this case the animals) around us. We communicate with events in our lives not just the people we talk to. Our thoughts, via the subtle energy that they transmit, are the language we use for this communication. Words let us schmooze people, hiding what we really feel and think about them. We can't lie with our energy. What we really think and feel is obvious to those who are sensitive, regardless of what we say.

Our subtle energy field constantly interacts with all that is. Everything in our world interacts with our subtle energy. Obviously some things, especially people, generate stronger reactions than do other sources. Our energy fields are a continuous series of complex attractions and repulsions, like molecules in a chemical soup, forming bonds and new compounds. These interactions determine events in our lives. Consequently, the world feeds back to us in many ways both physical and energetic according to the information in our subtle energy body.

We call this karma. Karma is not some exotic new age spiritual concept. It is a Sanskrit term meaning action/reaction. We set up the reaction with energy from our thoughts and actions. What we create with our energy is a direct reflection of our level of understanding and awareness. Regardless of whether our energetic communication to the cosmos is conscious or unconscious, we created the content of our consciousness and its ensuing manifestation.

Although there is no luck in the sense of events in our lives being random or chance occurrences, are we lucky in the sense that there is a divine purpose to the nature of order? Is there an underlying principle that moves all living things in the direction of perfection? Obviously this concept is inherent in any definition of learning, growth or truth. Seeing the truth of this is growth and it inevitably moves us toward perfection.

Synchronictiy

We have all been surprised by synchronicity. Was it chance you ended up sitting next to your future spouse at the lecture or were there other forces at work? Was it chance you asked her out? Did you ask because of her looks or the energetic vibe that you unconsciously received? All life is synchronous; it is a rich potpourri of interactive creative forces. The events in our lives are ordered as a result of the energetic information contained in this energy field. In other words, we create synchronicity.

If we follow this reasoning a little further we come to the realization that we, as all human beings, are responsible for whatever we create in our lives. Each and every thought and emotion has creative energy not just potential. It immediately goes to work shaping our next event. Will that next event be an illness? Will it be meeting a new friend or lover?

Many feel that the notion we are responsible for our illnesses is not fair. The difficulty in accepting this notion is that we are not very conscious of what we are doing that creates the events, illnesses and fortunes in our lives. It is true the word *responsible* implies conscious awareness of the causative factors. So it may not be the right word. At the very least, we need to realize that our thoughts and actions are at work shaping events in our lives long after we have gone to bed.

Louise Hay and others have helped many people discover that simply when we love ourselves and others we unconsciously create affirming events. When we hate ourselves and others we tend to create pain and misfortune. In *You Can Heal Your Life* the focus is on achieving this state through affirmations. However, a big question remains, to what extent does an affirmation such as "I approve of myself" change the energy of an underlying derogatory belief? What similarity does this have to faith? Is negation of the belief, seeing the falseness or arrogance in the derogatory belief, perhaps more effective at clearing the energy? Ultimately, when the negating is through what will remain? Trust perhaps?

Looking at how we create in our dreams, unencumbered with a body, we get a sense of how easy it is for spirit to create. While dreaming, we shift and move effortlessly from one scene or event to another. We are usually unaware of the thought or energy that created the shift. It is as if we are watching someone else's movie. In day-to-day physical form the same processes are at work just much more slowly, so we can study and learn from the cause and effect process.

Elementals—Its the Thought That Counts

Thoughts start energy moving at a fundamental or elemental level. These energy information packets or elementals have an affinity for similar energy. In subtle energy realms, like attracts like, and pulls people and events to it. It's very shocking and painful to have to take responsibility for our creation when we have no conscious notion that we did anything at all.

Even once we have a sense that we are creating our reality, it is still very frustrating. We are all used to thinking freely and believing that thoughts don't count, that actions alone are important. Wrong, wrong, wrong! Thoughts are actions and very powerful!

Elementals are created by our thoughts; they immediately go to work affecting the surrounding energy fields. The effect will be to attract similar energies to converge upon the elemental and you. These energies will have people associated with them. If the initial thought is anger directed at an angry person it will have the effect of drawing more anger into your personal space and consequently bathing your tissues and cells in it. This could be very unhealthy depending on how long you loiter in it. It will also draw other angry people into your life. This is a simplified picture as we all have many different emotions or energetic frequencies in our space at the same time.

Elementals also repulse energies, consequently keeping people and events away. What will happen if someone you want to date is sincerely sweet and loving while you are full of angry elementals? The chances of meeting this person will be diminished. If you do meet, there may be more repulsion than attraction depending on other energetic factors present. In many instances you didn't even have to say a word and your fate was sealed.

Have you been at a party where a person across the room stands out? Your eyes meet and you feel zapped, you get a little light-headed and flushed. Soon you are sharing your life stories and exchanging phone numbers. This is an example of elementals at work. It is common to find employees of a business who seem like they all came out of the same mold. They may look alike and their personalities are definitely alike. The group's elementals will always attract similar people to the organization. Bosses and personnel managers are often attracted to people who share their vibrations.

If the elemental is fear, other fearful people will be drawn to you reinforcing and fanning the flames of paranoia. Bathing every cell in the body with fearful vibrations causes stagnation in the energy system. This leads to a whole host of illnesses if stagnation remains in the body for any length of time.

Elemental thought forms or vibrations affect more than our health, they draw to us people and events. Thoughts of affluence and abundance may bring new job or investment opportunities. Dwelling in thoughts of not having enough will create situations of lack and need. What can we do about these thoughts and beliefs that write the scripts for our lives? See Chapter 11 - *Time Gone Awry, Change Just Happens*.

Energy is the music and language of the universe. It is the language by which the universe communicates with itself (us). It is the very essence of truth. Illness is just one form this music can take when we are in physical form. Our creations can take many forms that often put us in situations where we may develop abilities and talents that may be lacking.

Chapter 3

When you desire phenomena, you will get phenomena;
you do not get God.

—Peace Pilgrim

Disease as Signposts to Revelation

In addition to creating illness for growth we create illness because
we don't know any better. We go about life unaware that we are
attracting forces of deterioration. Developing our awareness when we
first find ourselves in a fresh young body is a bewildering experience. It is
made more confusing by inheriting a consciousness that is fraught with
misconceptions, half-truths, and false beliefs. As a result of these
misconceptions, we often lose track of our life purpose and deep interests.
Much of our life is spent in the pursuit of pleasure and respectability.
Consequently the true meaning and passion of life become clouded with
ethical shoulds and competition. There is no judgement here as all
experiences have something to teach us but the consequences are not
always pleasant.

Szent-Gyoergyi, Ida Rolf and others point out that in living
organisms, Form follows Function. Serious medical practitioners must
extend this idiom to include disease.

**Disease is an integral part of our form and it has a very important
function. Disease is not just something to be rid of or to be cut out
without understanding its wisdom. Disease is a communication
between body and spirit and vice versa.**

Its function is to make us aware of or dispel the misconceptions,
half-truths, and false beliefs that we hold. It is nature's communication
or consequence, and not punishment for the presence of rubbish in our
minds and bodies.

19

Have you ever journeyed to someplace new—maybe a vacation in a foreign country? You have no particular agenda other than to enjoy yourself. Perhaps you decide to go visit a historical site. You get directions from the locals and you are on your way. Some of the landmarks and junctions were subtle or poorly marked. Maybe an attraction beside the road caught your attention at the wrong moment and you missed your turn. Unaware, you confidently continue onward.

Soon, little clues appear that you are lost. Perhaps you round a turn and discover a town that isn't on the map. Confusion and doubt begin to creep into your head. Is the map out of date? Is this the right road? You continue on and more landmarks aren't consistent with the map. You stop and ask a stranger but you don't speak the language and it only adds to the confusion. The map shows a paved road and the one you are on suddenly turns to gravel. If you continue to ignore the signs and go farther in this direction, events become more foreboding; the gravel becomes dirt and continues to deteriorate. It starts to rain and you get stuck in the mud or you get a flat tire. Perhaps the engine dies. That familiar sinking feeling descends like a cloud, your desires are thwarted and you are unable to reach your goal.

Does it sound familiar? Is it similar to the way we journey through life? Looking at our illnesses as being incidents along life's way, we can see that we had a hand in their making. All too often we are inattentive to early warning signs. The early warning signs are subtle discomforts. Many of us are trained to ignore minor discomforts and pain. If we ignore these messages, the symptoms will soon begin to shout. If we are tough and stoic, we still ignore them. Eventually, they won't be overlooked and the body fails or collapses.

Our bodies are always trying to communicate with us. Sometimes we're distracted by other things or seduced by something interesting or we just choose not to look, but the signs are always there. Illness, discomfort, and good health are all a physical expression of the energy we embody. Even without disease, the body still provides us with a portrait of the energy within. Our posture, the lines on our face and hands, the 12 pulses, the way we walk and move all have something to tell us.

This portrait offers insight on our journey through life. The further off track we get the more serious the consequence or disease. Illness, disease, aches and pains, emotional disturbances, depression excessive joy, rage all are for the wise, signposts along the road of life. Just like signposts on the highway these signs let us know when we need to make a change, perhaps a new job, a divorce or we may just need to learn to speak our truth.

On the positive side "All roads lead to Rome" although some roads are more direct than others are. Guidance need not be painful; on the contrary intuition, joy, passion and our inner voice first guide us. Do we know how to listen? Are we in touch with the reasons for our particular birth? Usually the higher forces within us will create a blessing out of a tough situation, if we listen. Perhaps as we are fixing the flat and pulling the car out of the mud we get directions and information about a great out-of-the-way ruin or treasure. Was this the intent all along? Is there intent behind synchronicity?

The Drive in Living Matter to Perfect Itself

Disease aside for a moment, many people don't acknowledge a divine let alone a divine purpose. It is not necessary to believe in divine intent to see the interaction between subtle energy fields and the subsequent connection to illness. Even mere human observation changes experimental outcomes. This *wisdom* operates through subatomic subtle energy interaction. Subtle energy is also the medium of information by which the human aura operates.

Winner of two Nobel Prizes for scientific research, Albert Szent-Gyoergyi put forth in the paper *Drive in Living Matter to Perfect Itself* that there is wisdom operating in living organisms. In this paper he points out that to a biologist a carbon atom is just a carbon atom but to a nuclear physicist every carbon atom is unique. The atom is composed of subatomic particles that all have their uniqueness and unpredictability. As a result every atom has its own personality. Other studies have shown that this personality then behaves uniquely in the presence of other personalities.

When we alter the personality of the atom we alter the personality of the molecule. Affecting the personality of the molecule will change the company the molecule keeps. This affects our biochemical makeup which alters cellular, tissue, and organ function. The challenge is learning the language of subtle energy which is the language of subatomic particles.

The Meddler

Subtle energy is also the language of the modern healer. As we learn this new language, we begin manipulating and influencing these subtle energy systems, if for no other reason than curiosity. One danger inherent in this process is the tendency to micromanage events. Just as many people, encouraged by their doctors and advertisements, will reach for the aspirin bottle as soon as they get a headache, many healers will clear our discomforts as soon as we feel a twinge of pain. When we feel any uncomfortable foreign energy in our space we may want to remove it immediately. This foreign energy could feel like a pain in the neck, headache or bellyache. It could be an important vibration to experience with an important message or lesson.

If we don't look at what the issues are about before clearing the energy around a symptom, we will have to deal with a similar symptom again very soon. This principle applies equally to doctors, chiropractors, naturopaths, self-medicators, energy workers or any one in the business of treating symptoms. Before meddling in the patient's life and simply removing symptoms, there are questions the patient needs to consider, with the help of the practitioner. What message does this uncomfortable foreign energy have for the me? What is it trying to tell me about the direction of perfection? Why should I be thankful for this? What thoughts or actions brought this energy into my body?

Years of clinical experience teach the healer that **less is more**. In acupuncture using just a few points to bring the meridian system back to a balanced state is best. This sends a clear message resulting in a treatment that is easy for the body to assimilate.

In contrast, adjusting the pulse too minutely by stimulating many points makes the pulse hard and rapid (an undesirable state). The most desirable treatment for any illness is developing an insight into the wrong thinking or behavior that is the origin of the malady. Once this is achieved, very little stimulation to the energy system is needed to achieve balance.

Five Element acupuncture focuses treatment on the tonification of a root deficiency, promoting balance and enabling the body to heal without any direct removal of symptoms. It involves tonification of one or two points. Balancing the meridians enables the patient to gain insight into the cause of her problems. Clairvoyant readings can also reveal the root cause of a symptom and provide the education to clear the symptom in a natural way.

Clinical experience also teaches us that some energies are clearly stagnant. Such unhealthy energies need to be circulated immediately for the body to remain healthy or even alive. Other illnesses can hang out until the psycho-spiritual issues reveal themselves. The wisdom required to know the difference is the difficulty with energetic and psychic healing. It is also the beauty.

Healing is not a package, sold by multinational businesses; it is a process of self-exploration and self-understanding. Some illness requires emergency medical intervention at the physical, biochemical and meridian levels as well as the causal. The physical and biochemical options include drug, surgery, herbal or other treatments. Meridian level modalities balance the energy or Qi through acupuncture, shiatsu, Jin Shin Do or other forms of oriental medicine. The causal level includes the subtle energy associated with the mental/emotional body as well as spirit.

Healing is not achieved by applying a cookbook recipe to illnesses with the same name or symptom. Every patient and every illness, even if it bears the same diagnostic name, is unique. There is a unique set of circumstances, a unique cause, and a unique energy system and behind every illness a unique lesson. **Healing occurs when the lesson is learned, not when the symptoms are alleviated**.

> *There are two types of people who come to a Rolfer. One has what I so elegantly call a bellyache, and wants you to get that bellyache out. The other's ache is an overly absorbing recognition of the fact that he is unhappy. He is unwell, uneasy. He wants to know why, he wants to move on, and he wants to know more.*
>
> —Ida Rolf

The Art of Living

Getting healthy and staying healthy is an art. *It is the art of living.* The key ingredient is being in touch with our true passion, being on our path if you will. We all have an agenda, a life plan or path with specific lessons to learn. It takes great sensitivity to our inner emotional states so that we are guided down that road, our own unique highway of life. This sensitivity is fundamental to good health and the art of living. Again we have many desires for pleasure and security that dull our sensitivity to right living. This is not to say that indulgence in sensual pleasures is wrong but is it your path? The compulsion or the motive behind the choices is all-important and it is absolutely individual. Where do our priorities lie?

Some illness is due to neglect, overuse, exposure to the elements, and abuse. In modern times the most common form of abuse is inactivity and overeating. Few of us are sensitive to our body's demands and needs. All too often, performance becomes a priority and we sacrifice our bodies to get the job done. It matters little whether it is building a house or playing football. This is not to say that athletics abuses the body, but the potential is there.

Professional athletes have to push their bodies to the limit so they can have the experience as spirit of being a champion, summating Mt. Everest, or whatever it is they are seeking. An energetically healthy body is of course very resilient and can take a great deal of physical abuse. Yoga, oriental medicine, exercise and nutritional science provide us with much information we need to keep a healthy body.

There is a direct correlation between how healthy our energetic body is and the degree of abuse our physical body can take. If spirit is able to use the body for the purpose it intended, express its passions completely, in that fulfillment there is tremendous energy available. Not just available, but it has a different quality, it flows differently, smoother. If our energy is healthy, nutrition becomes a secondary factor in health. Food allergies are a result of toxic buildup of unhealthy energies in the subtle energy layers. Consequently, any deviation from a healthful diet for that individual is a form of abuse.

If we are healthy and listening to our bodies, we won't crave junk or convenience foods. Organizing our lives so that we can have time to prepare and eat healthful meals is part of the art of living. If we crave sweets then there is an imbalance in our life. What is the energy behind the craving? What thoughts or beliefs are at its origin? Most likely we are not getting enough sweet in our emotional life. What are the issues underlying this fact? All our cravings have a story to tell. Are we listening?

Even when healthy, being ill at ease is still a signpost giving us information about what works and what doesn't. When we experience a disease we must investigate the issues reflected in our choices. These decisions and attitudes created the energy patterns that led to the illness.

Chapter 4

The hardest thing about seeing the truth is seeing what a fool you have been.

—Buddhist Saying

The Growth Period

Some discomforts and ailments are merely spiritual growing pains. This category of bodily disease we call growth periods. It is more of a dis-ease than a classical disease. A growth period is the interval between change made as spirit and the consequent change in the body. For spirit, the change happens instantly. However, bodies need time and space to change. The growth period gives the body a chance to catch up to energetic changes made as spirit. Some practitioners refer to this healing reaction as a *healing crisis*. We did not create these illnesses for growth; rather they are a result of growth.

The energetic and informational field that surrounds our body controls our physiology. Our bodily tissues and cells are bathed in an aura of subtle energy. These energies determine the rate and type of metabolic activities that take place within them. Our cells and tissues get used to a particular vibratory bath. When a revelation takes place or when an issue has been understood, the energy field changes. This change in the energy bath is reflected in a change in our biochemistry. This creates a chain reaction; our glands secrete different amounts of hormones sending still another new message to the cells, tissues, and organs. Every cell is affected. When a change is made in one layer of energy it forces changes in the other layers, affecting our tissues and organs and how we feel in our bodies.

This change is healing, it is not always comfortable. More often than not it is uncomfortable. Growth periods may even be more uncomfortable than the disease but they are necessary and inevitable.

27

Colds, flus, depression, anxiety attacks, pulled muscles, twisted ankles can all be results of growth. Growth period discomforts will usually last only a few days. A clairvoyant reading can tell you what is behind this particular discomfort and help you move through it smoothly. Other growth periods are simply wonderful and ecstatic. This growth period may be experienced as just having a good day.

We did not create these illnesses to learn a profound lesson. Rather the message is that your body needs special consideration. The wise person pays attention to what the body demands to move through a growth period smoothly. Your body may want to eat special things or nothing at all. It may want sleep, exercise, dancing, hiking, walking, meditation, massages or a soak in a hot tub. Only your body can tell you what it needs. Again, the wise person attends to the body's needs, the numb ignores the body's demands and the fool resists them. Resisting the growth period and its physical or emotional discomfort will only prolong it. Resistance inhibits movement and movement is necessary to find a new easiness in the body.

The emotional reaction to the change can be quite intense. Although growth periods usually pass quickly one may want to seek help from a therapist or healer to move smoothly through these changes. Various types of therapies and energy work can help one move smoothly through growth periods. Some very helpful ones are acupuncture, Natural Force Healing, bodywork, Zero Balancing, running your energy, clairvoyant readings, and aura healings.

In the infinity of life where I am, all is perfect, whole and complete. I recognize my body as a good friend. Each cell in my body has Divine Intelligence. I listen to what it tells me, and know that its advice is valid. I am always safe, and divinely protected and guided I choose to be healthy and free all is well in my world.

—Louise Hay

Chapter 5

What we can't express runs our life.
                              —Unknown

Taking Responsibility for What We Create

Nothing makes us angrier than the notion that we are responsible for creating our situations in life, especially if we are sick. Hopefully, you are currently enjoying health and wealth so this concept can be reflected upon without resistance. Taking responsibility for our creations gives us the power and motivation that will make us effective at moving down the road to Wellville. It doesn't matter if it is a disease or wellness, a new job we love, or getting fired from one we didn't like, it is still our creation. Understanding how our thoughts and actions set us up for the end result can be tremendously empowering.

The movie, *The Postman*, featured a Pablo Naruda poem. The poem's main idea is that the world is a metaphor. The externally manifested world is indeed a metaphor for our own internal states, as our own collective internal states created it. While the world at large is a manifestation of our collective karma we create our own little world within it. A "shell hell" or shell heaven" if you will.

The realization that we create all the situations and events in our lives empowers us. This information gives us a handle on fear. With this realization our self-awareness grows and we become aware of the karma that comes with initiative and creative energy.

It is important to understand that our thoughts and feelings, guided by the beliefs implicit in them create our world, our reality. When we negate or eliminate the false beliefs in our conditioned consciousness, we become free to create in a conscious way. Moving from the old victim-based mentality to consciously creating your reality is tremendously freeing. This growth in and of itself will go a long way towards healing most diseases in the body.

On the down side, this is easier said than done. Most of us have tremendous resistance to looking at the beliefs creating our present situations. Many of the beliefs that are the basis for our actions were created in early childhood as the result of much pain and trauma. Questioning these formational experiences can be quite unsettling. Much of our belief system lies so deep within our psyche that we don't have a clue it's there. Much of the time we respond to events automatically, thought doesn't seem to be involved. These beliefs can range from racist attitudes, because we had mean neighbors of a particular race or believing that all women are loving goddesses, because our mother was. We don't go through a series of thought processes and evaluate each woman or person of this race, but it still can be a factor driving the beliefs that form our creations.

Overly self-critical attitudes can lead to creating from a place of self-hatred versus self-love. Combine this with a belief in good, bad and punishment and we begin to picture what type of situations we will be creating. Arthritis is one very likely scenario. The case study below is one of many similar stories.

> *94-year-old male. Retired utility company executive. Moderate to severe scoliosis with very pronounced rotation of the lumbar vertebrae. One kidney removed with much scarring around the area. Severe low back and leg pain. Heavily medicated with several strong pain killers, heart and kidney medications. His pain was intense despite the medications. Required injectable medications to sleep. Much dizziness and cloudy thinking. Withered and weakened right leg with a very limited range of motion. He could not sit through the intake interview without spasms, wincing and tears from the pain.*
>
> *Virtually pain free after eight acupuncture treatments— strength and coordination improved in his legs. He no longer needed his walker. Later, he missed a few weeks of treatments due to travel. He developed serious edema problems. The pain returned. A clairvoyant reading revealed a picture of him hitting and stabbing himself. He had many perfect pictures that he didn't live up to. His beliefs of not being good enough went all the way back to his childhood and were emphasized by his mother beating him. It was a*

very sobering experience to listen to a 94-year-old man bemoaning his mother's admonitions. After three acupuncture treatments the pain and edema were under control and he continued his pain medication just in case. The treatments were discontinued when he moved from his apartment into an assisted living situation.

A visit two years later revealed little change. He felt his productive life was over and he wanted to die. Wanting to be free of the pain he begged his "angels" to help him leave the body, to no avail. Again, a reading revealed that he was staying alive just to punish himself.

When we believe in good and bad or reward and punishment there are a multitude of ways we can punish ourselves. Louise Hay's book *You Can Heal Your Life* includes a list of mental patterns and the probable illnesses they create that range from acne and asthma to warts. She also suggests new thought patterns to heal the disease. As an example, she lists warts as little expressions of hate and a belief in ugliness. The subsequent affirmation, "I am the love and beauty of life in full expression" is the basis of the new thought pattern she advocates. It is an excellent list for practitioners to keep in mind as they work on patients. Ms. Hay suggests affirmations as a good way to alter current thought patterns.

There are other ways to make change that may be even more effective. Affirmations can have the effect of putting icing over a moldy cake. Clairvoyant explorations are often more effective at getting to the root of an issue. Once the lie in the belief has been exposed, the thought patterns will change effortlessly. The process of negating the underlying belief will be explored in depth in Section II.

By being energetically drawn to the time and place of birth, we choose what energetic influences we will be dealing with in our life. When we conceived of this birth we developed an agenda, a spiritual path if you will. We chose our parents and the geographical situations that would suit our situation and what we wanted to learn. We did not choose consciously in the sense we think of as having free choice in the body mentally picking this over that. Rather it is the nature of our spiritual energy and the information contained therein that makes our choice for us. A series of energetic attractions to potential parents and family members land us in a birth canal.

Once in a body we have no remembrance of what we came to explore and learn about. The nature of these influences and the type of growth they inspire can be derived from our Astrological Natal Birth Chart. The influences of the planets and stars set the stage for the underlying creation energies on the mental emotional level, (our personality). They get us started on our spiritual path. If our growth lesson revolves around experiencing lack and poverty, we are unlikely to manifest a winning lottery ticket no matter how hard we try. On the other hand, if your path is to learn about the great abundance and bounty in the universe, the winning lottery ticket may blow into your lap while you are waiting for a bus, you won't even have to buy it.

Healing or getting well is not something that is limited to the treatment room or doctor's office. We constantly create situations in our lives that force us to look and deal with the issues that make us sick. This is often done synchronously with others working out their issues with us. Life is just one big classroom and your state of wellness is your report card. The degree to which you are experience joy, wellness and sense of fulfillment can be one measure of the success of your creation.

Denial and the Life of the Victim

Denying responsibility for your creation (your life situation) requires resistance. Resistance to change is futile. You will eventually become what you resist. The nature of resistance is that the energy of whatever you are trying to resist sticks to you and you soon become that. You will soon vibrate at the vibration of whatever it is you were resisting. It doesn't matter whether it is your mom or another authority figure, you too will soon be assimilated. So deny and resist please, and you will soon understand the true nature of the victim mentality.

If we believe we are not responsible for what we create, then we must be lucky (insert your favorite noun) when we are the recipients of a windfall. When the result is not very pretty, then we are victims. It is interesting that the English language does not have a noun that is the opposite of victim. Is it that we like to take credit for working hard to bring about the windfall but want to deny a role in disaster?

Society has been in love with the idea of victim and punishment for thousands of years. Few beliefs have caused more pain, grief and disease. The mindset of the victim, while very popular, serves to confound our energy and starts us on a course of destructive action. The destructiveness of this internal movement unfolds in our relationships and in the larger social sphere.

If we are victims, it is that we are victims of our own consciousness and conditioning. A consciousness that lacks understanding of its own role in the creation process.

The courts overflow with victims demanding punishment for those who are *responsible for victimizing them*. In this punishment there is no justice, only vindictiveness and the desire to modify the behavior of the aggressor. While justice will forever remain elusive in the mind of the mortal, behavior modification meets with varying success but at what costs and to whom? The world religions have used blame and punishment to modify the behavior of societies for centuries and we are more violent than ever. What does this energy of blame and punishment create?

This external drama sets the stage for the victim to be victimized again, reinforcing the belief in good and bad. When victims fail to live up their own expectations or ethics, they consequently judge themselves as bad. This sends the message that punishment is in order so they are again mugged, swindled, hit their thumb with a hammer or are somehow victimized. The victims, not recognizing a self-fulfilling creation, once again go to court and start the process all over again. Ultimately it serves no one and is very costly to society as a whole. Watch the phenomenon in your own life.

A study published in the *British Medical Journal* found that bullies themselves were often victimized by other bullies more often than other children were. In the subtle energy realms, like energy attracts like energy. If we think that a person needs a beating because they are overbearing, guess who else gets beat up for the overstatements. Whenever we send an order out for someone, we should realize that we are making a duplicate order for ourselves.

Denying responsibility sets in motion a self-sustaining pattern of reactions and actions. Suffering for all is the result. The world could be a different place indeed if we understood how easy it is to change the patterns of suffering in our lives by changing our internal states. To take responsibility for our situations instead of denying our duplicity in the process is a giant step forward that will touch all humanity. Justice can only come through education. Justice can only exist before the next crime is committed, not after its occurrence.

Many profit from playing the victim card. It is an attempt to control others and get them to do what gives us pleasure. The victim controls interactions by taking advantage of the pity or compassion of others. The victim drama is an attempt to create order in our lives by controlling others and the external world.

Historically, belief in victimization is rooted in a very materialistic view of the world. That is like saying the cause of events in our lives is external to us. This results in a belief system that does not acknowledge spirit let alone its ability to create just by imagining. Accepting this belief in an external generated reality results in great fear and feelings of powerlessness.

Socially this has the effect of making us more controllable. Fear of Satan or fear of the police, it does not matter. In any case, we need to ask who benefits by the fostering of these notions? Who benefits from trying to control us in this way? What do they want?

Fear as, mentioned above, is the great Qi stopper. When our Qi stagnates, disease and ill health are sure to follow. It is the universe telling us we are not in harmony with the cosmos. The physical fear of being on the edge of a precipice is natural and necessary. However, the psychological fears from worries and anxieties can only exist if there is a belief based on a lie operating in our minds. In the absence of such negative beliefs, trust is the natural background state of beingness. Unfortunately, we commonly bury it beneath layers of false beliefs.

The planet is in the midst of a paradigm shift around the notion that we are victims, but few of us go willingly. The work is in making the shift in social awareness from one of victim consciousness to one of taking responsibility for our creations. That means we need to become observant of what we are thinking and thereby creating.

Getting and doing clairvoyant readings is a great way to develop awareness of these phenomena. In clairvoyant reading one can clearly see the origins of the effects she is currently experiencing. Clairvoyance in this context is merely using the faculties of our sixth chakra to translate the information contained in the energy surrounding an event, issue, or relationship. It is an ability that we can develop with the proper training.

Responsibility and the Child

Taking responsibility and making conscious choices is well and good for adults with the time and the mental acuity to do so. Our children are presented with quite a different situation. They come into the world physically and emotionally vulnerable. The infant is at the mercy of the adults around him. Are children not potential victims? The state of their energy field before birth has guided them to these parents and surroundings.

What learning and growth take place from abuse? Can abuse result in positive character development? Is abuse necessary for this development? Is it a karmic result from previous actions or previous lives? Would you abuse a child? What kind of situation would push you to child abuse? These are questions people have to answer for themselves.

The trauma the child experiences (including birth trauma) stays in the body for a lifetime unless much work takes place to heal and clear the damage. The following case study is an example of the healing many of us must do as adults to resolve the abuse issues we developed in childhood.

38-year-old female. Weak and thin pulses. History of much childhood physical and sexual abuses lasting into the teen years. Neck pain stemming from an injury in the shower; the shower nozzle popped off spraying a stream of water in her face causing her to fall backwards in the tub. Suffered debilitating pain for several months. She underwent surgery in which the upper cervical vertebrae were screwed and wired together. The surgeon believed the muscles and ligaments in the neck were too loose to stabilize the head. A year after the surgery, the pain was still intense, but better than before the surgery.

If the body was a car or machine, fixing a loose part to the frame with screws and bolts would certainly be appropriate but the body is not a car. It is a living dynamic bundle of tissues bathed in energy. Shattered bones from car accidents may need to be plated and screwed back together while they heal. Her's was not a bone problem; it was a soft tissue malady.

In this particular case the neck and upper back muscles, such as the levator scapulae and erector spinae, were rock hard. To enable movement of the head, compensation had to take place. The muscles and ligaments of the upper cervicals of the neck became hypermobile and over stretched to accommodate movement. A delicate situation. If a vertebrae popped out of position, the spinal cord or nerves could get pinched.

The treatments focused on treating the neck pain with acupuncture and moving core level energies with energetic techniques such as core integration—focused on the upper back. This relieved the neck pain in less than three months, with much improvement evident after the first treatment. The patient returned to work. The pulses remained weak and thin, even though they would improve after each treatment.

After about 15 months of treatment, the pulses greatly improved becoming more solid and full. The patient felt well enough to ride a jet ski. The energy in the thoracic muscles began to soften and move, not the muscles themselves but just the energy. In another month, the muscles themselves began to soften and move. The pulses continued to improve, becoming stronger and more balanced.

Soon the patient started releasing much anger and hostility, followed by nausea and a severe rash on her face and abdomen. These symptoms (Liver Wind to the practitioner of oriental medicine) signaled the release of old buried anger, and cleared dramatically with acupuncture (particularly Ken technique on Liver 3). A referral and visit to a M.D. ruled out appendicitis as the cause for tenderness in the lower right abdomen. The rash reappeared the following week. It was less severe than previously and cleared again with acupuncture. Finally, the muscles in her neck changed dramatically. The thoracic muscles softened greatly and the cervical muscles greatly increased in tension. At this point the screws and wires are doing more harm than good. They limit range of motion, continue to be locally tender and inhibit the natural flow of Qi or energy through the area.

Chapter 6

Eventually, everyone sits down to a banquet of consequences.
—Robert Louis Stevenson

Senority
The Art of Owning Your Own Space

The Divine Purpose of Physicality

We create as spirit to learn about the universe. As spirit we have the ability to create just by imagining things. It is just like the process in our dreams, where we have a thought in our mind and it plays itself out in imagery. It is more than just imagery, even in our dreams. The images have energy and emotional content. As in a dream, one scene often leads into another scene, with no continuity or apparent connection. In the spiritual dimensions, as in our dreams, the creation process happens so quickly, we appear out of control.

Spirit creates a body to learn and grow. Having a body is like learning to ride a bike with training wheels. Not that planet earth is the first stop on the evolution of the soul's journey but it could be. Being in a dense reality enables us to study certain phenomena at great depth. Incarnating in a body, with a dense vibration, slows the creation process down so we can study the cause and effect in relationship. A person who finds the learning process difficult might create a spiritual path involving science and learning about cause and effect. This person might even become a scientist and teach others how to learn about cause and effect.

Others may have mastered science and are ready to learn about the nature of beauty. They may become an artist or interior decorator.

We grow by developing a creation and learning from the results or consequences, and finding out what works and what doesn't. There are many levels to *something working*. Do we feel fulfilled and at peace? Was it a character building experience? Are we experiencing good health? If a physical creation such as a table, does it inspire awe with the beauty of its lines?

In-and-Out of the Body

We learn best when we are actually in the body, not just connected to it by an energetic cord. What does it mean to be in the body? Think of our spiritual or energetic body as a cloud of subtle energy and information that can change shape and split into different clouds, as do the water vapor clouds in the atmosphere. The spirit energy however is not blown about by wind rather it is moved about through affinity and energetic repulsions.

Our thoughts and those of others are a type of energy that will affect the cloud in this way. We can either have a lot or a little of this cloud within the parameters of the body. If this cloud (us) is in the body the information within it is available from which to create. If the cloud (cloud A) of information drifts away from the body and another cloud (cloud B) drifts into the body then the information in cloud B will influence the body. The ensuing creation will be based on cloud B's information. The consequent creation will not have much feedback information for cloud A about his own nature.

The Creation Game

We create from the energy present in our space. If we are going to learn about who we are, then we must have only our energy in our space. In everyday life this is seldom the case. Having only our spiritual energy in our body or *owning our own space* is not as easy as it sounds.

Many of us have wanted something only to be disappointed when it manifests. It's just not as satisfying as we imagined it would be. Perhaps we have even created an unbearable situation. Maybe someone works ten years to become a doctor and finds it is not the kind of healing she imagined. Now she is trapped by insurance companies and overhead expenses. Is it really a soul satisfying experience? Maybe the hypothetical person would be more fulfilled as a gardener or musician. What do we really want to create?

To put it very simply, we create our lives, the people in our lives, the events, and the energies we experience. We don't physically create people but we draw them to us by the attraction of our subtle energy fields and other karmic phenomenon. Our creations (our relationships) add yet another dimension to the energy in our space. Each new person and event has a new vibration which in turn puts a new spin on our reality. So pay attention to the company you keep and those you choose to be around.

Life is a very dynamic milieu, with the script being written as we go. Most of us are writing our scripts unconsciously because we react to events from our conditioning instead of responding with our creativity and wisdom. We let our conditioned thought patterns create for us. Creating meaningful change in these patterns is a most arduous task. Have you ever tried to change a habit? There are several types of energetic healing modalities we can use to assist us in this change: Natural Force Healing, acupuncture, Zero Balancing, clairvoyant readings and almost any kind of energetic treatment.

So, we create our lives from the energy and information in our space. We create the energy in our space from many sources. Foremost is our spiritual information. Thoughts and reactions to people and events in our lives, and the environmental setting also contribute a great deal. The earth's background energy along with music, architecture, and even furnishings of a room all influence the process. Everything has a vibration and consequently has the potential to influence our own vibration.

Some people are masters at creation and are little influenced by these energies. These masters are able to stay centered and maintain a focus on their path and what they intended to create with this birth. The novice is easily influenced and seduced by all the energies and information that surround him. The result often means confusion or being a pawn in someone else's creation game.

Seduction

Some energy initially feels seductive and very appealing. However, once in our space, it does not feel healthy or comfortable. The ensuing manifestations may be quite troublesome. The energy of lap dancing establishments may be a good example. The seductive energy of the dancers may feel good initially, but it could take days to get clear of the diminished feeling and irritating energies that accompany it. What do you think you would create with this energy in your space? What are the dancers creating? Who is using whom?

Some situations holding seductive appeal for us must be experienced over and over until we see they hold no real value. We may need to get completely familiar with it whether it be gambling, power tripping, or promiscuity. The results can be very unfortunate but learning isn't always easy.

Moment to moment awareness of the energetic conditions within and around us is key to owning our space. Without owning our space there is no responsibility in creation. Most of us are so focused on the material aspects of an event or interaction that we don't even notice the energy present. We are more concerned with whether we are going to benefit from a given event than we are about the quality of energetic textures and nuances that are present. Are we consciously aware of what we are focused on or are we just lost in the wanting? What is it that turns our clock, what do we want so badly that we lose our centeredness? Is it companions, sex, a good deal on a new car or house? What is it that can take us away from a loving vibration?

During any interaction there is always an energetic vibration present, usually it is a rich potpourri of vibrations. Even when interacting with a rock there are still vibrations present, especially if the rock is a crystal. Sometimes the energies descend upon us like a dark cloud. Other times they may lift us up so we feel like we are on a cloud. This energy contributes to our future creations.

Energies are drawn into our space by our thoughts, emotions, desires, and other people we encounter as we walk down the street. If the vibration doesn't find a resonance within us, it will pass on by. If the energy of someone on the street resonates with our own, then there will be an attraction. If we are an aggressive sort of person it will stick to us or invade our space. If we are vibrating with love and compassion then we will attract love and so on.

When we have many desires in our space it is very unlikely that we will manifest any of them. Rather we create confusion and become irritated. Commitment to one desire or goal will be most effective (providing it is in alignment with your spiritual purposes). **Purity and**

intensity of intention are key ingredients in focusing your energy for conscious creation.

Once this is mastered or at least understood, then one is confronted with the Aladdin lamp dilemma. If someone has three wishes, what is it that she would really want? What phenomena do you truly desire? What energies do you want in your space? Do you want the energies associated with lots of power, fame, wealth, and respectability? The fringe benefits associated with power, fame and wealth may look like responsibility, power struggles, harassment, or guilt for having so much when others do not.

As the picture of interconnectedness between issues and conflicting desires begins to emerge, our ability to keep a very clear and clean mental/emotional level diminishes. The mental controller becomes overwhelmed. If all goes well, the intellect comprehends the futility of the situation and the controller shuts down and you are once again free. The spirit is free to operate through the body without the overriding neuroses of the intellect. If the intellect just doesn't get it, a nervous breakdown or chronic fatigue may result. If the mental function is slow, the controller won't even notice and just keeps trying to get some satisfaction.

There are many other reasons for spirit to leave the body: physical pain, emotional pain, being new to the physical realm, confusion from conflicting desires, and foreign energy invasions. A well known example is the experience accident victims have of watching the crash scene while floating above the highway.

When spirit abandons the body, the result is feelings of loneliness. As a result of these foreign energies in our space, it gets very uncomfortable for us as spirit to be in the body. So we leave, and the body is on its own to manifest its creations.

Without the help of our spiritual energy to manifest, our bodies must effort in the physical realm to make things happen. Without spiritual assistance, we are less able to draw to us the people and events that make our creations appear like magic. This kind of struggle and strife wears out the body and usually ends in despair, depression, and loneliness. The body gets lonely for us as spirit and, thanks to our belief in externality, we look outward to other people, especially sexual partners, to fill the void.

Being

Our tissues, organs and cells all need the energy bath provided by our energy as spirit. Just as an automobile engine needs oil to run smoothly and for many miles, our bodies need the energy of our spirit to function smoothly over the long haul. One of the Yogi's purposes in doing pranayama (controlled breathing exercises) is to bring more of himself or his spirit energy called Prana into the body. It can be said that everything goes better for the body with our spirit in it.

There is a direct relationship between attentiveness and the amount of you or your Prana in the body. Likewise there is a direct relationship between spiritual growth and the ability to be attentive. **The key to being senior and owning your own space is to just simply *be*.** If the intellect is not busy clinging to attachments in the past or creating desires in future-time, then there is crisp attention. With awareness within and without we will be senior in our body. When we are minding our own business, not judging others but seeing them through eyes of compassion, we will own our space.

Chapter 7

As far as your self-control goes, as far goes your freedom.
—Maria Ebner Von Eschenbach

The Banquet of Consequences

We often joke about someone who must be possessed without believing it to actually be true. The subjects of these comments are usually people who are inordinately passionate or obsessed with something that is not in their best interest. Possession and exorcisms have generated attention in the movies and elsewhere in the media. Understandably, the sensational nature of this phenomenon makes good copy. In contrast, western medical circles have ignored the concept and prefer to focus on medications for those who act a bit odd. Possession has been treated as a medical condition in oriental medicine from ancient times to the present. Clinical experience has shown possession to be more than sensational fiction.

In Christian cultures, the possessing entity was usually the ultimate evil archetype—Satan or other lesser demons. The movies or novels rarely portray the possessing entities to be harmless lost souls or well meaning guides, which they often are. It makes no difference whether evil or well meaning, having another entity's energy system in your space and in your body creates emotional and physical havoc. Ill health will soon follow.

We have all experienced someone else's energy in our space or aura. We attempt to influence and control others in this way. The difference between having someone's energy in your space and a possession is basically a matter of degree. It is not an all or nothing phenomenon.

Beings without bodies have been known to hop in an empty model and take it for a joy ride. Like walking down the street and finding a convertible with the top down and keys in the ignition, it can be quite tempting. When we are not fully in our bodies this is the situation we create. By virtue of being connected to our bodies via the "silver cord," an energetic link, we have seniority in the body. Being senior means we have the right and responsibility to remove foreign energies and entities from our space. To do so we have to be aware of their presence and ask them to leave. If they refuse, psychic and acupuncture techniques will remove these guests.

The stage for intruders is set when we have made the environment inside our bodies uncomfortable with unhealthy thoughts and emotions. Much of our spiritual energy leaves and a sense of loneliness and desperation sets in. When we as spirit leave, we've opened the door for a foreign energy or entity to enter.

Foreign energies usually enter through the transmedium channels located in the neck and shoulders. Once in, the neck and shoulders feel tight and the head seems foggy and achy. Other symptoms include blurry vision, clouded eyes (as the eyes are the windows to the soul or spirit), attention deficit disorders, high level of stress and angst, and difficulty establishing connections with others. Some people will notice very little if anything, and may just pass it off as a stiff neck.

Physiologically, every aspect of metabolism is affected; the whole system is stressed. According to the oriental medicine system of diagnosis, it produces a Yin deficient type of condition. Yin deficiency creates thirst, irritability, excess heat and rapid pulse. Physically manifested illnesses are all over the board; possession can be behind any disorder. It can lead to eczema, heart disease, carpal tunnel, fibromyalgia, arthritis, etc. Every body has different weaknesses and the energy of every entity is unique. The degree of possession in every individual is variable.

There are three principles that underlie owning your own space:

1. If we don't own our space, someone else will.

2. Others don't take our space. We give our space away.

3. We are senior in our bodies; others must give way.

Often, we as spirit have made contracts with these beings to run our bodies. Life may be just too intense or overwhelming and we needed a break. As years pass, the interloping entity gets quite comfortable and can be rather reluctant to leave. This is when a practitioner familiar in these matters is quite helpful. Again the consequences on the performance and health of the body can be quite severe. Bodies function best on their own spiritual energy not the energy of other entities.

The Casual Interloper

We all experience energy invasion on a more casual level. It is just someone else's energy getting in our space. These invasions are usually other people trying to control or influence us.

The most common is a person hitting on us sexually. One person running sexual energy in our space makes us predisposed to engaging in intimate conversation and physical acts. If we respond by running sexual energy in return, and the vibrations are compatible, the relationship may spiral into euphoria. We might say there is chemistry between us. It is that energetic high or rush we associate with falling in love. It usually has little to do with love, and more to do with trying to get a connection externally instead of energizing the body with our own energy.

Another type of interloper is not so pleasant, the angry competitive sort that we often run into in the workplace. They may appear to be meek and mild and have everything under control. They will get in your space with a different kind of energy that makes you feel like you have been beaten up. This is an attempt to make us timid so they can manipulate and control us.

You can experience this invasion by stepping in front of others, waiting in the checkout line, at the grocery store. Most likely, you will have a few of the people behind you silently invade your space. Stoic people who say little will probably get in your space. You will likely experience some uncomfortable symptoms, such as headache, pain in the neck, and foggy head. If they speak up and tell you "go to the back of the line bub!" then the energetic invasion probably won't happen.

An important fact to remember is that these invasions are of our own making to bring our attention to some issue or belief that we need to look at. We need to ask—why are we bringing this energy into our space? These casual daily occurrences can create illness especially if the energy remains in your system for a long period of time. A long-standing psychic battle with a spouse or child can create serious illness; with symptoms, as for possession, all over the board. If the energy is just present for a few hours or days the reaction may only be a headache and tight neck and shoulders.

Thirty-year-old female with severe environmental sensitivity. Allergies to most foods, and most everything. Lived in a "clean" house and confined to it for the most part. She was not a possession case in the normal sense. She was not taken over by one entity. She had much difficulty with boundaries, emotionally and psychically. Her blue envelope was full of little "nipples" or conduits. These nipples enabled entities mostly without bodies, but also individuals with bodies to connect and draw energy from her system. These conduits also let in all kinds of foreign energies and being depleted she was unable to fight them off, so her body suffered. The envelope was repaired with energetic healing techniques, and much improvement was observed. The underlying issues of feeling inadequate remained. The conduits would continue to reappear until the underlying self-esteem issue was resolved.

The Guru Experience

The guru experience occurs when a guru or teacher takes over someone's space. It is a specific type of possession. The devotee's commitment and involvement in the community will determine the degree of takeover.

When the body has been abandoned, the loneliness gives rise to an external search for comfort. Becoming a member of spiritual community begins to look like a good fix. The intellect may learn valuable lessons for later use.

In the ashram, people give up their power and bodies to a guru. The guru controls multiple bodies, and enjoys the benefits and power of many bodies. The spirits actually connected to the bodies hang out in limbo—dazed and confused. The result is that the rest of the people (their empty bodies) in the group or cult will have an experience of oneness, as the guru's energy (spirit) is in them all. They all have the same spirit energy in them, giving rise to the sensation of oneness. Not realizing that the oneness was the guru's energy at one with their own energy, the devotees believe that they have achieved oneness with God. This so-called peak experience is a good hook to deeper devotion. It becomes a bit of a let down when they leave the group and re-enter society and that oneness is no longer there.

The guru experience is an interesting form of communism; the body now acts and creates from the guru's information. The inherent trial and error process by which we learn from our creations is thus short-circuited. However, one of the things a person may need to learn is that being part of a cult is usually empty and unsatisfying in the end. This trial and error learning is what one could call **Spiritual Science**.

Cults

Possession and the cult in western society are very similar to possession and the guru in eastern cultures. The word cult is another one of those terms heavily laden with emotional charge. The first thing many of us think of when we hear the word *cult* is devil worship, weird religious groups, mass suicides such as Jonestown, and aliens returning to the mother ship. Webster's defines cult as a system of worship of a deity, great devotion to some idea, or thing, a sect. Sect is further defined as a group having a common leader or a distinctive doctrine, one of the organized bodies of Christians. A cult member is someone with the energy of the leader or leaders in his or her space.

This leader often exudes great charisma. The word *charisma* comes from Greek meaning gift. Webster's defines *charisma* as—a quality of extraordinary spiritual power attributed to a person capable of eliciting popular support in the direction of human affairs. In other words, a cult usually has as a leader someone with the gift for getting their energy in other people's bodies. The leader influences the way members think and act, so that members profess belief in the leader's doctrine or dogma, very similar to the guru. Cult leaders also inspire the group to follow edicts that may seem outrageous to the ordinary person.

The bizarre part is that the leader or leaders do not have to have a body. Often churches and cults have a group of out-of-body entities that are responsible for transfering the energy of the cult into the space of the churchgoers or cult members. This is especially the case with Pagan or Wiccan covens, where a witch without a body presides over the coven and manipulates the energy in the group members. Some of these energies can feel very good and loving, even euphoric. At other times, they can be intensely painful, especially if the entity is trying to influence you in a negative way.

This implies that these entities are guides and in a way they are. What kind of mischief might they be guiding you into? Is the guidance coming from wisdom or a more perverted place? Perhaps power, or control? Respectful guides do not get in our space and most importantly do not prevent us from being in our bodies.

Remember that we take a body to learn and to grow. We learn most when we are creating with our own energy and information. Are we learning about ourselves if we (the body) are creating from someone else's information? Once again, giving up our body to the guru, the church, or the coven is giving up an oppotunity for growth and development.

The energy around organized religions finds its way into the space of its memebers. However, few invade to the degree that it becomes a cult. Very involved participants, such as priests or nuns, experience greater invasions than the casual parishioner. One often enters these organizations with the idea that she is giving her life to God but in reality it turns out to be more giving it up to the church and its hierarchy.

Many of the new Christian sects, the born-agains and new age fundamentalists with the charismatic leaders, have crossed the boundary into the realm of true cults. Members believe the euphoric peaceful feeling they are experiencing is actually Christ. In reality, it is the energy of the group. The group may be channeling the vibaration of an entity who does not have a body. This energy actually affects your perception and the way you think. It can create a zombie-like effect with glassy or veiled eyes, similar to being on drugs. In some cases, the transmedium channels (the entry points for our spiritual energy) of these individuals are "psychically-surgically" altered to allow the presence of these energies. Permanent damage to the body is possible over time.

So, if it feels like bliss, what's the problem? Again we take a body to learn and grow and this is only possible if we are operating from our own spiritual energy. Our body is designed to run with our energy in it. Therefore, for it to stay healthy it needs to have as much of our own spiritual energy in the body as possible. Otherwise, cancer and many other illnesses will be much more likely.

You and your body may not like what the alien energies create, a creation that you ultimately will have to live with. Often individuals awaken in twenty or thirty years, unhappy with the position they find themselves in. It often looks like bankruptcy, emotionally, financially, or healthwise. In any case, their lives don't turn out they way they would like.

Who is responsible? Are you going to blame the person, group or church that used you or are you going to take responsibility for giving up your space, power and authority? Whose life turns out the way they would like? Have your life choices been created by you as spirit? At least you have learned a great deal, and your body is most likely healthier.

It is easy for those skilled in reading and running energetic vibrations to recognize the real Christ vibration as well as many other wonderful vibrations, such as love and grace, but it takes a discerning mind and some experience to know the difference. Many cults can fill your space with energies that produce the experience of euphoria. This euphoria may make you think you are communing with Christ or God when in reality you are not.

If we are indeed able to bring the Christ vibration into our body then the question becomes--why? What purpose does this vibration serve? Do we want Christ in our space 24 hours a day or just for a few minutes? Why do we want this vibration for our own? Is the misery so great that we don't want to create from our own energy? These questions are not to suggest we shouldn't invite Christ but are intended to faciliate and exploration of the phenomena. It is healthy to understand the why and when if having Christ in our space is indeed something we want or need to do. Is there a compassion vibration that exists independently of the Christ vibration? Is compassion something we can generate as spirit ourselves?

Spiritually when we are not in a body, we learn and mature less effectively, the body functions poorly, and is prone to disease. Professional athletes will always perform better when they are in the body. They will be able to run faster, jump higher, and have greater agility. **Not being in the body could be the best way to define a wasted life**.

The Alien Possession

The alien possession is not a very common occurrence but has come up in clinical practice on several occasions. Theoretically it doesn't make a lot of sense but in the reality of clinical practice it can't be ignored. If you ignore what you think you are seeing just because it seems too weird or bizarre you are doing your patient a great disservice. Oriental medicine teaches techniques to deal with alien possession!

The alien possession is basically a parasitic being or group of beings from another reality. These beings connect to the subject via energetic cords in order to steal energy. The possessed subject often has an agreement to receive something in return from these entities. A clairvoyant reading could help determine the nature and reason for the contract.

I doubt possessions are worth the energy cost to the subject, but it is his or her decision. The aliens often tap the individual in the back in order to drain the Kidney Qi. The kidneys are the center of the will, and these individuals usually have no will to fight back or throw the aliens out of their space. This is a trick also employed by the pagan witches that predates Christianity. The old goddess religions would use this technique on men, later turning them into zombie-like slaves until time for sacrificial ceremonies.

In any case, possessed individuals usually have many health problems. Some form of exorcism is necessary for the patient to improve significantly. Exorcisms can be performed either psychically or with acupuncture. The psychic will probably be most effective at addressing the multiple problems affecting the energy system.

Section II

Self-Healing
The Fast Track to Wellville

You wake up; you look out of the window, and say to yourself, "Oh, awful rain." Or "It is a marvelous day but too hot" — you have started! So at that moment when you look out of the window, don't say a word; not suppressing words but simply realizing that by saying, "What a lovely morning", or "A horrible day", the brain has started. But if you watch, looking out of the window and not saying a word to yourself — which does not mean you suppress the word — just observing without the activity of the brain rushing in, there you have the clue, there you have the key. When the old brain does not respond, there is the quality of the new brain coming into being. You can observe the mountains, the river, the valleys, the shadows, the lovely trees and the marvelous clouds full of light beyond the mountains – You can look without word, without comparing.

But it becomes much more difficult when you look at another person; there already you have established images. But just to observe! You will see when you so observe, when you see clearly, that action becomes extraordinarily vital; it becomes a complete action that is not carried over to the next minute.
—J. Krishnamurti

Chapter 8

Be fiery, cold one, so heat can come.
Endure rough surfaces that smooth you.
—Jelaluddin Rumi

Rent Asunder
The Legacy Revisited

At birth we inherit a consciousness that sees a world of separate individuals instead of a colony of cooperative relatives. It is this notion that has set people against one another in a competitive, empire building frenzy that continues to the present day. It is not that we aren't individuals but it is the spin that is put on the concept. The spin is composed of a myriad of subtle nuances held deep within our conditioned brain. The brain's message, in brief, is that we need to fear life and protect ourselves, not trust. We need to get others before they get us. The legacy of our ancestors passes to us subtly through concepts and beliefs implicit in language as we learned to speak. At a very early age we adopt beliefs about the nature of the world by watching others in relationship around us. From these beliefs we form a concept of the world and our place in it.

An unfortunate aspect of the world view we inherit is its fragmented nature—resulting in over dependence on thought for information about the world. Thought is a tool with a job to do. The nature of this tool, thought, is discriminative in function. It separates one object from another. It *recognizes* groups of characteristics whether they are part of a physical object, a personality or a sensation within the body. Thought also separates and groups items based on a comparison of features. If two things are not exactly alike, thought can recognize the difference. Some subtle differences in objects or phenomena cannot be distinguished without special instruments. For example, the temperatures at which two liquids freeze requires a thermometer. Obviously, we all differ in our abilities to perform these tasks.

If we assume certain constants that define the parameters of particular phenomena, we can make predictions. In engineering, we use statistical probabilities to predict that a given roof truss will be adequate to hold up a roof, assuming a maximum snow load or wind stress. Even in this case, it becomes a matter of probability not certainty, which is all that is required in construction, or nothing would ever get built.

Familiarity enhances our ability to perform complex tasks, such as finding our way out of a maze. Familiarity can also lead to what psychologists call *functional fixation*. We become functionally fixated when we have learned a method for performing a particular task. The task changes while our technique does not. Another technique may be easier and more effective but we cannot see beyond the one we have learned. Medicine, for example, continues to treat diseases with drugs when an energetic treatment would be more effective and with no *side effects*.

Human thought, through its ability to distinguish characteristics and organize them into a new creation, makes life in a body a marvelous thing. Like any tool, thought should be used properly. The danger of thought is of getting lost in the labyrinths of our concepts and losing sight of the whole.

Thought does not stop at making just one level of distinction between objects, people, or phenomenon. Thought separates them further into categories. We all do this with relationships; we separate people in our lives into categories. Those we know well and those we barely know. Those we trust and those we do not trust. Those who have something we can gain from and those who appear to have nothing to offer us. Those who have brought us pleasure and those who have brought us pain.

There are many, many levels to our discriminatory processes, and one category can often conflict with another leaving us with a confused messy consciousness. Like engineers we try to make predictions, as to whom we want to share time and energy with. We make thousands of judgements each day all based on our past experiences. In any personal relationship we must discern a preference from millions of qualities. How do we choose which are important?

This choosing is the fodder for much gossip and water cooler conversation. The possible qualities we can use for comparison are so vast that the few we end up with can be considered arbitrary or at least so capricious as to make the whole process farcical. It would be something to laugh at except that the consequences are profound indeed. This constant comparing and judging leave us with a residue of separateness. The resultant separation and isolation can make the situation quite tragic. Indeed, the separation may be only psychological or it may manifest into physical isolation but the impact on our energy system and consequently our health can be devastating. On a lighter note it is all learning.

Divine Purpose or Wrong Turn?

Does this separative aspect to our consciousness have a divine purpose or is it a product of thought gone awry? Perhaps the real story has elements of both—the body has built-in purposeful limitations and thought has gone awry.

The chakras are configured to regulate the quantity of energy available to our electrical and nervous system. This energy regulation allows us to maintain the feeling of being separate individuals. When all the issues associated with this state of being are clearly understood, the energy regulator called Kundalini unwinds and allows a transformation in the energy system to take place enabling transcendental experience. The regulator is called Kundalini because it resembles coiled earrings women wore in India. It comes from the Sanskrit word kundali meaning earring. Kundalini regulates the flow of Qi, Prana, or life force into the central channel or sushumna.

The function of energy flow through the central channel is to circumvent certain structural limitations built into the chakras to keep us in a time based physical reality. Without these limitations the human system has access to information in other dimensions. Without this transcendental experience to connect us to the reality of the divine, we commonly become overly dependent on thought. We soon ascribe undue certainty and validity to the product of the thinker. Consciousness has a habit of identifying with the thinker believing it to be much more than a tool. The problems associated with this subtle distinction will become apparent in subsequent chapters.

In addition to the limitations placed on our energy system by Kundalini, spirit will often create physical limitations in the body (e.g., illness, low I.Q., lack of physical beauty or great physical beauty, etc.) that enable or even force the individual to learn particular lessons. However, one needs to be careful in ascribing every limitation or difficulty we face as an intentional creation of spirit. Many of the difficulties we face are just part of the process of learning—learning about creation, learning about being and learning about relationships.

Chapter 9

*The foolish reject what they see, not what they think;
the wise reject what they think, not what they see.*
—Huang Po, Zen Master

Clairvoyance

Clairvoyance simply means to see clearly. It is the process of making the information that is available to us as spirit available to our everyday conscious mind. Information is contained within subtle energy fields. All information has a vibration, not entirely unlike radio waves. The human body is the most sensitive instrument for sensing this vibration. It is probably only a matter of time before someone invents the clairvoyant computer that can pick up and translate thought form vibrations into text. The defense department has used psychics for this in the past.

Clairvoyance is the process of converting the vibration into information that can be apprehended by the brain (ordinary consciousness). This process takes place in the sixth chakra where the information that exists as vibration is translated into pictures. *Clairaudience* translates the vibration into sound and it occurs in the fifth chakra. For example, you may "hear" somebody speaking to you without him uttering a word. He may be quite shocked when you respond to what he only thought. *Clairsentience* translates the vibration into physical sensation in the second chakra. You will feel the emotions of others as if they were your own.

When the body becomes sensitive to subtle energy and uses its clairvoyant functions to translate the information then **energy becomes the universal language**. It doesn't matter if the person you are reading speaks French or Chinese; you can determine the person's intentions toward you. You may not be able to understand her directions to the Louvre but you can tell whether she is angry, or loving, in a hurry, or

57

about to do you bodily harm, and many other things as well.

Of course, a lot of this can be attributed to reading the person's body language. We often supplement the cues we get from a person's body language with the information we are receiving clairvoyantly. Bringing the issue closer to home, how often has your husband, wife, or roommate been irritated with you but not said a word? He pretends everything is fine but you know he can't hide those little thoughts. You can feel his irritation. You are feeling his energy in your space. If he communicates his irritation openly you may not feel anything. If he tries to hide it or suppress it, the emotional energy will come out anyway. The energy of his emotions will get into your space, usually via your neck and shoulder area. If you resist, it will linger and become more of a problem.

An Everlasting Imprint

The implications of this are absolutely phenomenal. When reading a person's energy there are no distortions, no lies can be told. Since energy can never be destroyed, it leaves a permanent record of every thought and activity. There would be no more fighting over biblical interpretations or distortions presented in history books. You can go to a historic ruin and read the energy and see and feel what took place there. It adds a new dimension to vacationing in historic areas. In a courtroom the jury could read the energy of the defendant and determine her guilt or innocence.

Like any new skill there is a period of development where one learns to trust the pictures and his ability to interpret them. Nearly anyone can learn. The first step is listening and becoming sensitive to one's own being. A capable teacher is essential, as there is much to learn. It is important to be able to discern the source of energy of which you are reading and to protect oneself from unhealthy energies.

Of course our sensitivity can be dulled. In most of us it has been blunted to a great degree. The body becomes insensitive from excessive living--too much noise, too much heavy food, too much wine and booze, too much partying and so on. We become sensitive or dull depending on how we care for ourselves. There is no magic prescription. Everyone has individual needs. So we must listen to the demands of our bodies to be sensitive to the energy and information around us.

To remain insensitive is irresponsible. How can we respond if we are not aware of the information bombarding us? Even if we are aware of it, an intelligent response demands that we interpret what we are feeling, seeing, and hearing. This interpretation is like learning a new language—the language of energy. As in learning any new language, a language teacher is helpful, especially at first.

Discernment

The self-healing process can only start if we are truly willing to look at ourselves. Looking at ourselves will be most useful if we can look from *nonjudgment* and with *neutrality*. We see others more easily than we see ourselves. It is harder for us to suspend judgement on ourselves than it is on someone else.

The beauty of clairvoyance is partly its ability to sidestep the pitfalls of traditional self-reflection. Most of our "ordinary" perceptions are not only colored and distorted by our self-interest, but also by our defensiveness. In doing clairvoyant readings on others we are also looking at ourselves. We all share the same consciousness and problems but in a different mix. When we see our issues in others we get the learning and understanding without the defensiveness.

We take defensive postures when we are incomplete and insecure in our level of understanding. This usually stops exploration in its tracks. If we are honest with ourselves we will see that we subtly and quickly judge everything. Everything gets reduced to: I like this or I don't like this, this is beneficial or this is harmful, this is support or this is a threat and so on.

Discernment is necessary but judgement needs to be kept on a leash. Judgement is out to kill like a rabid dog, while discernment is how we recognize those signposts on the road of life. Simply, does it feel like love or does it feel like competition? **Discernment** is the product of **clairvoyance,** while **judgment** is the product of **intellect**. The intellect compares a given thing, person or event to its perfect pictures and ethics. Discernment is what we learn as spirit from meditating on what we create. It is the process of applying what we learned from asking ourselves how it felt to have been the creator of a particular thing or event. Judgement is a habitual often, automatic response of the brain to almost any stimulation.

The beginning of meditation is the choiceless vigilance of this process. The clairvoyance takes the judgement and distortion of the conditioned intellect out of the process of self-reflection. It also enables us to look at others from a neutral viewpoint without the competitiveness of ego. Looking from neutral is a process of adjusting the energy levels of the chakras and learning to look from the sixth chakra. It is a matter of trusting your pictures instead of your thoughts or what someone else wants you to think.

There is an old Buddhist saying: "The hardest thing about seeing the truth is seeing what a fool you have been." In other words, if you are being a fool you will find out in a very matter-of-fact way. It is very difficult to be led astray if you use your clairvoyance, especially where new age spiritual matters are concerned. There are only too many well-meaning individuals ready to take us down the garden path, often at great expense. While reading the rest of this section on self healing, keep in mind that **being able to look and operate in daily life from neutrality and nonjudgment are prerequisites for self-healing**.

Fortune-Tellers and Psychics

Looking at spiritual information clairvoyantly is no different from the process a psychic or medical intuitive may use. The term psychic comes from the Greek word *psychikos* which means of the soul or life, a person sensitive to nonphysical forces. In modern parlance psychics have been associated with fortune-telling and doing future-time prediction. Little is heard of the psychics used for spying by large corporations and the defense department, but it goes on as a matter of daily business. Police departments have used psychics to help solve various crimes. It is merely the ability to tune into the subtle energy forms produced by our thoughts and actions.

Clairvoyance can be used for future-time predictions but this raises serious questions about the reader's responsibility. When a clairvoyant looks at a future-time event he sees one possible future. Once that picture has been looked at, the energy around the event changes. So what had been the most probable future will not be the most probable any more.

A reading about a future-time event can make us loony or sick with worry. We begin second-guessing how to achieve or avoid that future, again changing both the present-time and future-time energy. It is one thing if a clairvoyant wants to look at his own future but another when a client with little understanding of what she is asking for gets a reading.

A reading of the present-time energy around the person and her present life situation will help her much more in deciding what she wants to create than reading a possible future outcome. What is sorely lacking in most of our lives is a true understanding of who we are and why are we doing what we are doing right now. We all have the ability to see the truth of who we are by using our clairvoyance in a responsible manner. We have all the information we need to answer these questions, it is just a matter of learning how to look. Once we see, we have no choice but to be responsible.

Chapter 10

The Myth of Becoming
The Great Generator of Sorrow

Security is mostly a superstition. It does not exist in Nature, nor do the children of men as a whole experience it. Avoiding danger is no safer in the long run than outright exposure. Life is either a daring adventure or nothing at all.
—Helen Keller

One of the things we all share regardless of culture is the myth of becoming. That is the belief that we can psychologically become better and hence more secure through effort. This belief indicates a failure in society's ability to understand the process of how we change. Our misguided attempts at improvement take the form of imitating an ideal. Striving to become like our ideal, our heroes—what is wrong with that? It takes us out of present time and invalidates who we are, two major factors in disease.

On the surface we all want to be the best we can be. When we look closely at the phenomenon of becoming, we find that it is not about self-improvement at all, but about fear. It is the fear of being invalidated. Ironically, it is the desire for the ideal and subsequent invalidation that starts the process—a process that never ends. This lack of understanding is responsible for our personal suffering as well as the woes of the world.

Let's look closely at why we want to become better or even the best. If you are a world class athlete it can mean lots of money and adulation. This is not the becoming of which I speak. Becoming better at golf or tennis is a matter of training. We get into trouble if we apply the same process to the psychological arena. If we want to use effort to become less angry and more loving gradually, then we are deluded. Training isn't going to produce results. (See Chapter 11 *Time Gone Awry, Change Just Happens.*)

If we look deeply at our motives, we will find that we think becoming better or perfect will make us more secure. Secure in the sense that everything in the future will turn out to be good—with more pleasure, more respect, more control, and more power. The prevailing belief is that if we behave in a certain way, we will have a better chance of getting what we want. Most of us have a concept defining that *ideal* behavior. To conform to that ideal picture we suppress some behaviors and emotions while imitating others. So what is wrong with this picture? Let's slowly go over it again.

Invalidation and the Ideal

Intellectually each individual has a picture of what he or she has to be in order to succeed in getting what they want in life. This perfect picture or ideal is unique to each individual. Inevitably following from this perfect picture is the efforting or struggle to achieve or mimic the ideal. The process of conforming to this idealized image can have only one outcome—the **invalidation of who we actually are**. Not only do we make ourselves try to fit the idealized picture, we then try to make everyone else in our lives fit into our perfect picture, our perfect world. This invalidates others, and the battles and conflicts begin.

Invalidating others and ourselves with perfect pictures is the *Generator of Sorrow and Suffering*. Invalidation is more painful than it sounds. Those of us who had strict parents still hold physical and emotional memories of much abuse and invalidation. The trauma and abuse that we experienced when we fell short of our parents' perfect pictures made us feel as if we were going to die. Children depend on their parents for life. If the parent disapproves of the child and withholds support, the child may literally die. This traumatic experience is the birth of the fear of death.

As adults, at a subtle, below-the-surface level, we continue to fear we will die if we don't live up to our own perfect pictures. Even if we measure up to our own perfect pictures, someone is sure to point out our failures according to his ideals. We experience sorrow and suffering because we associate invalidation with the fear of death.

The process of psychologically or intellectually becoming safe through imitating perfect pictures actually is the process of *becoming* insecure. "Becoming" is a vicious cycle because the more we intellectually seek security, the more perfect pictures we generate. And the more perfect pictures we generate, the more we invalidate ourselves. These invalidations make us feel as if we are going to die. Hence we become more insecure. Looking for safety we generate more, perhaps different, idealized plans and perfect pictures. After 50 years of this cycle we wear ourselves out and may look forward to the grave.

> *A 70-year old patient came in one day, reflecting on his life. He felt like a failure. I said, "Get real you must be worth millions of dollars." He said, "Fifty-four million dollars to be precise, but my brother is worth over a 100 million."*

The myth is the belief that you can become safe or secure, through becoming wealthy or esteemed. You can't satisfy the demands of your own perfect pictures. You will always need one more piece of property, one more lover, one more sale, one more victory, one more friend.

Perfect pictures lead to comparisons. Comparisons generally make us feel inadequate, especially when we compare ourselves to the ideal. The brain habitually compares and habitually invalidates. What does it take to break a habit?

Imitating the ideal is an age-old legacy passed on by previous generations of parents and all those who came before us. Avoiding this inheritance is difficult because it happens at an early age. However, we are responsible for continuing it and propagating perfect pictures. We are also responsible for buying into the resulting invalidation of others and ourselves.

The consequence of continued invalidation is believing that we are no good, that we are undeserving of the *harvest*. In reality, abundance is readily available.

Let's knit some of these concepts together. As spirit we create our reality. This creation process is based on what we believe about the world and ourselves. What do you think is created from a belief that you are undeserving? At the very least, it probably won't be a fine, sweet, happy time! How do we reconcile the millionaire's failure attitude with his ability to create 54 million dollars? What might his life path be? What might his natal chart look like?

Chapter 11

It seems to me such common sense to begin with "what is".
—J. Krishnamurti

Time Gone Awry
Change Just Happens

Psychological and behavioral changes happen instantly as a result of an insight. We don't become incrementally better people through effort as we do in sports. While as spirit, change happens instantly, physical bodies require time to change. In order for the intellect to proceed with the process of becoming, that is imitating perfect pictures, it must create psychological time.

Psychological time is a lie, a sleight-of-hand conjuring trick, created by the brain. The brain erroneously associates the concept of physical or clock time, created when we move from point A to B, with psychological movements of consciousness. This is an illusion. Psychological change happens instantly in *present time*. A flash of insight imparts understanding and you are a different person. Your behavior will be irrevocably changed. This spiritual growth is very real healing for the body.

In golf or tennis, we can practice our strokes to train our muscles and become incrementally better over time. Conversely if we are violent and we want to be non-violent, practice is silly. At any given time you are either violent or you're not violent. There is no I am violent today and I will be moderately violent tomorrow and then less violent the week after. There is no tomorrow or next week psychologically, only the now the "what is." The next week is an imaginary construct. There are no muscles to gradually strengthen in control of violence. A little violent is still violent. Either you are manipulating your world with force or you are not.

A little or a lot of force it is the same psychological movement. There is no poor stroking of love like a poor stroke of the ball. There is no love muscle to incrementally improve. Change as spirit happens instantly. Bodies take time and effort to change.

Chapter 12

...fear is the non-acceptance of what is.
—J. Krishnamurti

Control vs. Creation
The Great Generator of Suffering

Invalidation, and comparing ourselves to perfect pictures, leaves a residue of inadequacy (see Chapter 10). We try to resolve this through damage control, to become secure. We want control of ourselves and our behavior as well as the behavior of others and our surroundings. Unfortunately, we frequently use dysfunctional control techniques.

These control techniques have as their basis a belief in scientific materialism. Cause is seen as material or external to spirit. Biological science doesn't recognize spirit, spirit energy or the subtle vibrations contained in information. Presuming that our lives are materially driven makes us think we change through effort.

The techniques we use to control the situation through efforting when interacting with others fall into four categories. These control dramas, as delineated by James Redfield in *The Celestine Prophecy*, are the interrogator, the intimidator, the aloof persona, and the victim.

The *interrogator* controls interaction with a barrage of questions, forcing others to think about the subjects and conclusions the interrogator is comfortable with or has interest in. The *intimidator* uses sheer presence and authority to dominate and control others. The *aloof* person stays above it all—nothing is ever wrong and there is no emotional involvement. The *victim* controls interactions by demanding sympathy. *Poor me* I am having such a difficult life. My dog died today and my mother is being evicted and she is going to have to come live with me, my employer is going out of business and so on.

The *martyr*, a special kind of the victim, gains control by doing so much for others that they can't complain about anything. Martyrs also use *guilt trips* to make others do their bidding. A talented individual juggles all four dramas, matching them to the person and situation at hand.

Control dramas often appear effective. We gain control and get what we think we want. In reality, they create dysfunctional relationships and are counterproductive. In the big picture, nonresistance to what is actually taking place is the beginning of creating real peace, harmony and good health in our lives.

Chapter 13

Just spread out a mat
For reclining quite flat
When thoughts tied to a bed
Like a sick man growing worse.
All karma will cease
And all fancies disperse.
　　　　　　　—Ch'ing Ming

The Process of Becoming (Whacko)

Becoming secure through the pursuit of the ideal is the basis for human suffering. The apple in Adam and Eve's garden is an early appearance of this dilemma. The process of becoming inevitably leads to heartache and violence. We wage war within ourselves at the very least and often extend the violence toward others. It is a process that we engage in over and over again in the course of a day. This process, over the years, wears down our bodies and bathes us in a variety of unhealthy energies. Becoming, as outlined below, is really the foundation for our suffering, illness and premature aging.

Different people have different strategies for controlling themselves, their environment, the people and the situations around them. However, all strategies share an underlying theme—a common formula. The process is common to all humanity regardless of race or culture. The steps involved in the process of becoming have been organized into the pyramid below.

The pyramid can be looked at either on its base or upside down. Looking at it from top to bottom, the progression begins with perfect pictures and progresses to ethics, competition and finally violence. If we turn it upside down, the psychological processes underlying a **violent** society are obvious. Becoming whacko is the actual outcome of the process. Becoming secure is the motivation for the process.

The Nine Steps to Becoming (Whacko)

1. **Perfect Pictures and Pain Pictures**—invalidate our reality.

2. **Ethics**—based on perfect pictures, the root of a corrupt morality.

3. **Judgement**—comparison of our ethics to behavior.

4. **Invalidation**—effect of judgement.

5. **Resistance**—resisting the comparison and judgements of others. You become what you resist.

6. **Efforting**—imitation of the ideal, empire building.

7. **Competition**—envy, jealously, hatred, destroys anything you try to create, toxic.

8. **Taking Responsibility for Others**—judging others political action, laws, punishment, destroys relationships.

9. **Whacking and Violence**—speaks for itself, but includes political action, wars, creating chaos, self hatred.

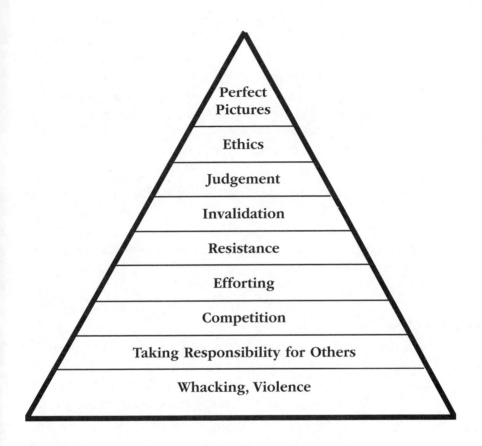

Pyramid of Becoming

Exploring each step in the process will only have meaning when we see the process in ourselves. Seeing the process intellectually and in those around us may be a first step, but it will not bring about the change that will empower our lives. Becoming whacko is not something somebody else is doing; it is the basis of daily life for each one of us. It is business as usual; it enables a state of chaos and is counter to us all moving into a mature state of creation.

Perfect Pictures

A *Perfect Picture* is an idealized mental image. It is a *should*: who we should be, what we should have, who others should be, what others should have, what others should act like, what the world should be, etc. This should be self-explanatory, pun intended. We all have core beliefs of what we think will make everything in our lives turn out good and pleasurable. In other words it is that which will make us secure. Our concept of security is composed of a conglomeration of perfect pictures. Perfect pictures are also the beginning of *desire*.

Perfect pictures are the basis for ethics. Ethics are the basis for more perfect pictures. This doesn't mean that we don't struggle to be a great carpenter, painter, or writer. It just means that comparing ourselves to an idealized picture is invalidating. Remember that our external world is based on and reflects the mental world within us. Consequently, we will create a world or reality reinforcing that invalidation. Ideals or perfect pictures invalidate our reality; they are the source of much self-flagellation. This sets the stage for an existence full of punishment in the physical world.

Pain pictures are a key component in the formation of a perfect picture. Our past wounds and hurts form our library of pain pictures. In order to avoid pain, much energy goes into creating a perfect reality. That is, a reality where there will be no recurrence of these painful events. We might think of this as seeking security. This is the most common state of the human mind, like aircraft in a permanent holding pattern over the airport.

It may be helpful to look at how a pain picture is formed or what puts pain in the **pain picture**. Mix one part perfect picture with a pinch of comparison. Add one self-image and viola, **instant invalidation** or pain. Remember that as children we associated validation from our parents with physical survival. The result being, invalidation makes us feel as if we are going to die. In this way, we were conditioned to avoid pain and pursue pleasure.

The perfect picture often becomes an unshakable belief in what would make us happy and content. Comparing perfect pictures to possible and probable scenarios of the future creates either enthusiasm or anxiety. Enthusiasm, if the perfect picture appears likely, and anxiety or depression if achieving our goal looks futile. If we come up with a *plan*, like a new job or relocation that may enable us to achieve our goal, we get enthusiastic. If the goal seems out of reach or we can't formulate a plan, we become depressed.

Thought moves through time, comparing its collection of past pleasurable and painful events. From this we formulate a perfect picture. In other words, we create our perfect pictures based upon our conditioning. It is important to always remember that whatever pictures you form in your mind, it is not the way things *actually* are, but they will nevertheless create a *reality* for you. If we foresee pain pictures coming down the road, then the anxiety intensifies. This anxiety leads to step three, **resistance**, and all the rest of the steps on the pyramid. Resistance is the beginning of manipulation (*the plan*) of people and events in an attempt to alter events in favor of avoiding the pain and realizing the pleasure.

Recognizing that there is a perfect picture behind nearly every thought is the beginning of meditation and a return to health and sanity.

Ethics

The dictionary defines ethics as a treatise of moral conduct. Morals, according to Webster's dictionary, are established principles of right and wrong behavior. These principles, obviously, are perfect pictures and will invalidate anyone they meet. Then again, if we are in spiritual competition the object of the game is to invalidate anyone we meet.

Debatably, ethics have been an effective way to guide proper conduct and control society. This begs the question—proper conduct according to whom? Whose perfect pictures are we adopting? The church, the society, the gay subculture, the environmentalists, the media, the business community, parents, peers or others. We all carry around with us a set of ethics, more rigid and defined in some of us than in others but nonetheless a set of rules. Rules about behavior based on our conditioning and other peoples' information with its inherent contradictions invalidating every one it touches.

All ethics have one thing in common; they are based on perfect pictures. The perfect pictures are based on arbitrary criteria developed into a belief according to our conditioning. Just as no two minutes are the same, no two situations are the same, even though externally they appear identical. No set of criteria for passing judgment can ever be all encompassing and consequently right action cannot be prescribed.

Ethics are clearly a body/intellectual concept, created consciously or unconsciously to control others and ourselves. Ethics generate much guilt that is essentially self-invalidation. Ethics prevent right action, they do not create it. By making the intellect senior to spirit we confuse who and what we are about. Spirit has no ethics. Spirit learns what works and what doesn't from all action, that is the value of creating. In short, stop trying to be *good* and you will learn much more about yourself and the nature of reality. In this way spirit is always moving in the direction of perfecting itself. This is not to say there shouldn't be consequences for heinous social acts. There always will be consequences, but beware of the self-righteous lawmaker.

Now that we know what ethics are, let us look at some of the consequences. If we feel we know what right behavior is, then we feel justified in judging and invalidating others and ourselves. Thus we are creating guilt, conflict, and chaos in our personal lives. Ethics is the weapon of choice for the spiritual competitor, the controlling parent, monarch or church. It is a poisoned arrow, inflicting a wound that decays slowly from the inside, until the whole being is crippled. Here we already have the basis for disease a psychosocial phenomena creating energy eddies and imbalances leading to disease.

Judgement and Invalidation

Judgement is simply comparing and applying ethics and perfect pictures to our behavior. We apply our own ethics to our behavior or to someone else's behavior. Likewise, someone else uses ethics and perfect pictures to judge us. The inevitable result is invalidation. Even if we compare favorably, if our behavior meets or exceeds our ethics and perfect pictures, it invalidates our uniqueness as spirit. An initial feeling of validation soon becomes the burden of conformity.

Judgement is a very powerful tool for social control but crushes our uniqueness as spirit. For example, the grading system in our schools destroys the A student as well as the underachiever by bending them to the mold with positive reinforcement. In some instances the A grades may reflect a student's spiritual nature. The student will be encouraged to deliver the same product. But next time, will it still be the same free expression of his nature? Grades may be an inevitable part of public education but the important thing is to understand what the process is still doing to our way of being in the world. It sets up comparison as a legitimate way of relating to each other and sets the stage for invalidation or being disrespected. Being judged and invalidated lead to the next step— resistance.

Resistance

We usually recognize resistance as defensiveness. When you feel defensive, look for the accompanying perfect picture or judgement that you experienced. Then look at why you feel defensive or resistant to the issue.

The perfect picture may be your own creation or a *gift* from someone else. Perfect pictures can be conveyed to us using overt comparisons, very subtly or just implied. You may be walking down the street with a friend who comments about another's sloppy attire. Because you sometimes dress in a similar style, you apply the judgement to yourself. We do this often without consciously thinking about it. It is not uncommon for one statement to have four or five perfect pictures hidden in it.

It takes a very clear and attentive mind to remain nonresistant in the face of invalidation. If you resist, you will become that which you resist. You will assimilate the mannerisms, beliefs and ways of operating from the culture or subculture you resist. Resistance triggers a very sticky vibration in your energy system. This vibration also makes your aura sticky. The energy of those you resist will stick to you, filling your aura and becoming your vibration.

Resistance is rejecting all that is not part of our perfect pictures. For example, resistance to your mother's perfect pictures, values and ethics allows them to stick to you. Soon you will begin vibrating at her vibration. The vibration of her values and information will become yours. Just as we resist the perfect pictures sent our way, we resist people and those aspects of others and ourselves that don't fit our perfect pictures. If your ideal world consists of all blondes then you will have resistance to all nonblondes. The more you resist, dislike or disapprove the more intense the stickiness. Finally, you are vibrating at the same rate and acting just like the person or value you worked so hard to resist.

There are many ways to resist: escape, denial, defensiveness, aversion, condemnation and so on. All can lead to illness depending on how stubborn and rigid the resistance. The type of discomfort or disease depends on the length of time the resistance has been present, degree of stagnation, other disease causing elements as well as the individual's overall strength.

Are we doomed? Is there a way out? The way out is simply to see the falseness in the perfect picture you are creating or resisting. When this is understood, compassion is the vibration that will replace the resistance. Whereas resistance acts like glue, compassion is the energetic equivalent of Teflon®, nothing sticks to it. Nonresistance is always the way out at any point in the becoming process. Resistance only prolongs the journey and creates chaos.

Efforting

Efforting is the energy spent making our reality fit the perfect pictures—an ever-elusive proposition. Efforting is a body concept, e.g., the physical effort necessary to climb a hill. As spirit we have the ability to create and change without effort. But if we're dissatisfied with our creation, with what the universe is providing, we often force the issue. Efforting is like the proverbial *pushing the river*. Trying to change the momentum of the universe is a good clue that something is out of alignment within us.

Efforting is something that is second nature to us, we no longer think about it consciously. We are usually so wrapped up in it that we have no perspective from which to view it. Perhaps the easiest way to see it is by looking at the various ways in which we try to control our interactions with other people. In our relationships, our efforting takes the form four basic control dramas (Chapter 12 - Control vs. Creation). We use these techniques to make a situation conform to our pictures of what will bring pleasure or security. These little numbers or trips we run on people usually start in childhood. By the time we are adults they are second nature and operate without our conscious intention. The control dramas are ways in which we found that as children we could get what we thought we wanted. If nothing else, we sought the accompanying attention and the energy that goes along with it.

Creating is as easy as imagining a new job. Change is as easy as seeing the folly in a particular course of action. Efforting is an advanced stage of resistance and it is folly, similar to spinning your wheels when you're stuck in sand, it only digs the hole deeper.

Competition

Competition is listed here as the fifth step in the process. It depicts the stage where we are actively competing and running that vibration of energy at someone or in response to someone.

Competition is a special case of possession. Specifically, it is the desire to possess superiority over another. This desire is born of the insecurity derived from invalidation and a separative view of the world. It is the basis for empire building and imperialism. There is nothing in this book more important than understanding the phenomenon of competition and seeing how it operates in your daily life. If you understand competition, then love and the key to the universe can be yours. If you don't understand competition, it will run or ruin your life.

Competing for survival, food and shelter on the planet has helped us develop strong bodies and energy systems through evolution. Competition on the physical or body level is a necessary thing. What would games be without competition? Competition spurs us on to do things we would not normally be physically capable of doing. It gives us the incentive to build strength and develop our potential. Many feel the strong bodies we developed through competition over the last fifty thousand or so years are necessary to handle the increased stress from the intensity of shifting energies. This stress is expected to intensify as the planet moves into its next step in global spiritual evolution.

Although competition in the past may have served a purpose on the planet, it is now like a runaway train. It has an unstoppable life of its own. Competition is everywhere: in the home, the office, our romantic relationships, schools, churches, recreation. You name it, competition is there. The saddest part is that very few are even aware of their own competitiveness. When new students are asked whom they compete most with, commonly four out of six respond that they don't compete.

The intellect is extremely keen at denying and hiding our selfish competitive nature. The first fork on the road to Wellville has a sign— to the left is the town of *Denial* and to the right is the town of *Self-awareness*. Which is the shorter route?

If we are to make any change in our competitive nature we must first accept the fact that, yes, we are indeed competitive. In fact, the whole **process of becoming is basically one of competition**. A seminar recently put forth the notion that the root of all evil was the desire to possess. As discussed above, the desire to possess starts with perfect pictures. I guess that makes the formation of perfect pictures the root of all evil. Although a perfect picture is harmless until we compare it to what is. Does that make comparison the root of evil? Perhaps?

Competition and its best competitors are esteemed and rewarded in almost all avenues of life. Top athletes make more money than some CEOs of large corporations and they produce only entertainment for those who enjoy watching competitive games. There is nothing wrong with physical competition on the court or ballfield. When we leave competition on the court or ballfield, there is no problem. The problems start when we combine our sense of self-worth with how well we performed compared to our opponents. In this way, competition spreads into the psychological and spiritual arenas.

If we take a closer look at this process, we see at first glance that it is enormously validating to make 25 million dollars a year as an athlete. It is even more validating to make more than your fellow athletes do. Then there are the trophies and awards. For most of us money does play a large role in determining our self-worth. So when we compare our 25 thousand to that 25 million we feel like we made a wrong turn. We form perfect pictures from our idols. The idols themselves could not live up to these idealized images, yet we compare ourselves and try to imitate them. When we compare our actual lives to these perfect pictures of success, we feel invalidated.

The comparison even robs the decorated hero of their uniqueness as spirit. The adulation and rewards have the effect of directing the individual's behavior in the direction of conforming to the public's values and expectations.

It doesn't matter whether it is in response to a particular individual, subconsciously responding to media advertising or we are simply trying to become respectable. Comparing what we have to a perfect picture or someone else still breeds competition and still creates chaos, leaving a residue of cosmic debris.

As spirit we have our own uniqueness—we do what we do better than anyone else. We all have a niche and inherent value. In the big picture, comparison doesn't mean a thing. Comparisons are based on criteria developed through our conditioning process. The criteria we use to make these comparisons are capricious at best and essentially arbitrary. To compete comes from the Latin *competere* meaning to seek. If we look at ourselves closely when we compete we will see that what we are seeking through competition is **validation and security**.

It is a rare person indeed who participates in an activity to simply strive to see what he and his body are capable of and are truly untouched by validation and accolade. In seeking validation through competition and comparison, we invite the more advanced stages of the competition disease—**envy, jealousy** and finally **hatred**. Now add groups of people into the equation and we have all the ingredients for politics and a recipe for war. Remember that if we have to rationalize what we do, it is not love, and that underneath every rationalization is an underlying need to compete. Without competition, esteem and wealth can still happen, providing it is your spiritual path.

Taking Responsibility for Others' Creations

Taking responsibility for others covers everything from *mother knows best* to political actions to the western medical philosophies. When we see a struggling friend, we want to give advice or share recent insights. Many parents have their child's career and future mapped out before he is through grammar school. The medical doctors make many decisions for us regarding drugs and surgeries and use their authority to convince us to go along. The politicians regulate many substances and activities they see as irresponsible and harmful to society. Some of these things may be necessary, but it is still invalidating and will breed resentment in some. Like a parent telling a daughter she must be home by ten o'clock. The message is that you are not mature, intelligent, or responsible enough to make your own choices.

It is always easier to see dysfunctional behaviors in others before we see them in ourselves. When we learn something new or have an insight, we apply it to someone else first. Isn't it natural for us to want to make everything better for others? Of course, we would eventually apply it to ourselves. The opportunity just presented itself in someone else's life first.

Giving unsolicited advice, validation or praise, passing legislation are some of the ways in which we take responsibility for someone else, to take responsibility for another's healing. Each invalidates the other person, sending the messages: "You're not managing your life correctly. I'm more competent than you are, so do it my way." Praise is superficially justified, but still sends the message that the giver knows more than the receiver. Our motivation derives from a need to feel better about ourselves. We're uncomfortable looking at somebody else's pain. Fixing things, offering advice or solutions is usually motivated by a need to ease our own discomfort.

Parents learn that forcing wisdom on their children can invalidate, leading to rebelliousness and other unpleasant reactions. The Grecian teacher Socrates sought to avoid invalidation by asking the right questions. Adroit questioning enables the wise to impart understanding while respecting the listener's responsibility for grasping and using the insight.

When tempted to meddle or give advice, it is prudent to ask ourselves a few questions. What criteria or ethics did we use to make this assessment, this judgement? What are we resisting? Do we see the perfect pictures involved? Are we willing to justify punishment or whacking (the next topic) for those who resist our meddling?

Spirit takes a body to learn and grow. We learn and grow from all our creations. We all are learning about different things, at different rates, and in different ways. All paths lead to God but some may take longer to get there, perhaps a few more lifetimes. Imparting wisdom by asking the right question or providing insight when appropriate can be an act of compassion and can shorten the journey and prevent suffering. Providing insight, when someone needs to solve the problem for herself, is invalidating and lead to conflict.

Seeing the consequence of taking responsibility for others brings an end to judgment. Without judgment, a true compassion will have a chance to flower for oneself as well as others. Action born of compassion will not be part of this movement of controlling and becoming. There will be no urge to take responsibility for the creation of another. Instead, we will share understanding in a manner that is empowering instead of invalidating.

Whacking, Violence

Whacking is a technique of psychically throwing energy at another person's aura. The whack usually smarts a bit and can be disorienting, until you find out where it is coming from. If you are hanging from the edge of a cliff where no one can see you, whacking is a good way to get someone's attention. Whacking as a weapon to punish or modify the behavior of others is as inappropriate as any other form of violence.

Violence is the culmination of the becoming process. Look at the pyramid turned upside down to see that it is not so much a nine step process as it is a psychological movement of violence broken down into nine steps. We do not consciously go through these nine steps in the moments before we are violent. The first six or seven steps could be sitting in our psyche for many years. We apply them in an instant at the right time when an opportunity arises. We don't always follow the process to the conclusion of physical violence but we go through the first seven steps every day.

The process of becoming is the formula that underlies social behavior, as we now know it. It is not the mental state of only a few felons and psychos. It is an almost constant process in everyone's mind. It is one thing we share the world over and will be with us for most of our lives. It is not something one can simply will away.

Some whackers are able to disguise their whacking so it appears socially acceptable. They can beat you up and still appear to be sweet loving beings. A well-executed guilt trip will make you think you deserve the abuse. We all need edification, but does anyone need to be whacked? A common defense is that the beating was for the victim's own good, to teach him a lesson. Perhaps? It may also be a lack of creativity. Many use innuendo and sarcasm in public, and save whacking for those with whom they are closest. The more we deny the presence of this subtle violence or deny that this behavior is violent, the more it will run our lives.

Violence can be controlled and modified with will and intention but it can never be eliminated with will. It only ends when the process of becoming ends. It is not something to fix by beating ourselves up. On the contrary, the way out is to make the process of becoming our best friend. Watch its every movement; get to know it intimately. Once totally understood, it will no longer be the force driving the operation of society.

Although fear and trust are not mentioned in the nine steps, fear is an important ingredient. Fear is generated once we form a perfect picture and it's accompanying desire. Fear arises when we speculate on all that can frustrate our desire for pleasure or security. Fear then becomes the fuel that propels us through the rest of the process. Trust is the water that can put the fire out.

Chapter 14

Beyond Becoming

almost anybody can learn to think or believe or know.
but not a single human being can be taught to be. why?
because whenever you think or you believe or you know,
you are a lot of other people; but the moment you are being,
you're nobody but yourself.
to be nobody but yourself – in a world which is doing its best,
night and day, to make you everybody else –means to fight the hardest battle
which any human being can fight,
and never stop fighting…
does this sound dismal?
it isn't. it's the most wonderful life on earth.

—e.e. cummings

Getting Free—There is Nothing Like Unbecoming

Getting free of the process of becoming is as easy as seeing that you create your own reality. It's as easy as perceiving that events in our external world are drawn to us by the condition of our mental, emotional and spiritual being. We change our life by changing our internal state thereby changing the energy we radiate. This energetic shift causes change in the outer world around us. Real change in our internal state happens instantly with insight or a flash of knowing.

Intellectually, this is relatively easy to understand. However, intellectual understanding rarely translates into behavioral changes. Most often, our behavior is automatic and habitually follows the nine steps above. Changing a habit becomes a difficult task when the rest of the world reinforces the old pattern in every moment. Moving from becoming to nonbecoming requires diligent vigilance of this whacko process in our own minds. Even with an insight into the falseness of becoming (whacko), it is necessary to trust this new information in the light of new threats (comparisons to the ideal).

To consciously create requires learning how to trust our own information and then to act from that information. Clairvoyant reading is a tremendous tool for putting us in touch with our own information. Reading others develops our ability to trust our pictures, enabling us to gather and trust our own information.

Once we understand that judgement and the process of becoming lead only to violence (and its nuances), we can either ignore it and numb ourselves to our resistance or let people be free. This often feels as if we are letting the vulgar get away with being jerks. Edification requires more than simple condemnation. The world's religions are still struggling with this concept. When we let others be free, we then free ourselves to give voice and expression to our own unique spirit. This expression often involves some form of education of those we now let be free.

This process of becoming consumes great quantities of our energy, leaving us very depleted and with an even stronger drive for *becoming better*. Even if we receive great quantities of validation from others, it won't run in our energy system. This verbal validation is like white sugar, with its empty calories, that rob us of vital energy. Consequently, no matter how good we are at competing in the whacko process, it results in a net loss of vital energy.

Love

Does love come from within or from external sources? Frequently, the more we feel unloved, and invalidated, the more we seek validation from others. This is an expected reaction with a mind that is used to thinking in material terms—what is real and substantive comes from outside us. Therefore, love comes from someone else. Is it clear that we feel unloved because we compare ourselves to our perfect pictures and the pictures of others and not because others don't love us? Validation or seeking energy from someone else is the beginning of competition and several steps on our way to violence. Clearly validation and competition are not love. To experience love we must be free of this cycle.

When the perfect pictures we have about ourselves stop, the validation/invalidation we seek stops and the energy loss stops. We become receptive to self-validation, and have affinity for our own beauty and uniqueness. Affinity or love is the great sense of joy at the mere presence of the beauty of someone's existence, be it your's or another's. The vibration of affinity will fill our being. When our reservoirs are filled and overflowing, this energy will naturally overflow into the world around us, splashing on others.

Chapter 15

Meditation is the total release of energy.
—J. Krishnamurti

Cosmic Debris

Humans store experiences as information in their auras and energy systems. Cosmic debris is the residue left by a messy consciousness, especially the waste products from the process of becoming. Residues include stagnant or suppressed emotions, traumas, invalidating ethics and perfect pictures, energies out of present time, thoughtform conglomerates, elementals and anything we resist. Over time, the build up of cosmic debris in our energy system leads to stagnation and blocks our flow of energy. The resulting stagnation weighs us down and slows our energetic vibration.

This stored information has an energetic vibration that includes a broad spectrum of colors, just like electromagnetic vibrations of the visible light spectrum. Different information has a different vibration and hence a different color. The colors can be seen clairvoyantly and have even been photographed. Clairvoyants learn to interpret the information contained in the colors they see. Some vibrations allow debris to accumulate at a faster rate. Other vibrations, such as gold and love, act like a slippery shield, allowing debris to slide off of us.

Our cells and tissues need to be bathed in fresh clean energy to stay happy and healthy, like water from a clear mountain stream refreshing all who drink from it. Energy fouled with debris like a swamp, leads to health problems. Uncleared debris attracts more debris until our energetic bodies are engulfed. The physical and mental effects are responsible for many degenerative diseases, particularly arthritis. By the time we are seventy, we could be walking (if we are still able) piles of cosmic trash.

This debris pile is created by our thoughts. These are thoughts that are out-of-sync with cosmic harmony or truth, particularly fearful competitive and abusive thoughts. Thought not only creates energy, but it attracts energy to it. Thought invites energy into our personal space. Thoughts are "me centered" snapshots of the world around us. Like a snapshot, the thought is never able to capture the whole; it is always an interpretation. This interpretation is egocentric as it is based upon the individual's experience and/or conditioning.

The instinctive response to this buildup of muck in our energy system is denial. We ignore the subtle beginnings of the buildup. Few of us have the skills or understanding to treat it. Taking analgesics, muscle relaxing medications and other painkillers do not address the energetic cause. The discomfort may be minimized by medications, but the fouled energy is still present and affects our metabolism and health. Social circumstances often demand stoicism so we continue to perform when we feel emotionally out of sorts, achy, or stiff. Avoiding discomfort is instinctive. We will want to move from this discomfort to a more perfect state so the brain goes to work, first creating the vision of what it wants and how to get it.

For most of us, a pill is the first thought—quick and easy. Is this the right tool for the job? Cosmic debris removal, according to natural laws, is both more effective and educational than biochemical doctoring. An epiphany or insight usually follows the release of energy that is associated with the illness. Previously we learned that measurement and comparison are inherent in the nine steps to becoming. What we really become in that process is violent and clogged with debris.

Concepts are like photographs, they are two-dimensional representations of multidimensional objects, distorted by the lens, filters and the aperture setting of the camera. Our concepts are interpretations of what is happening in the world through our filters of conditioning and the nine steps to becoming.

Some concepts may be a closer to actuality than others, but all are off the mark. Seeing the truth of this is what makes self-righteousness totally absurd. The awareness that the concept or the words in our head are not the thing, not actuality, is the beginning of meditation.

Having established that concepts are never truth or actuality, concepts do have energy and create effects or karma in our world. We can follow the nine steps to becoming and carry around the debris we create or we can stop trying to be better than, faster than, richer than and create beauty in our own lives independent of what others may be doing.

Meditation is the awareness of the limited nature of thought as it is happening. Meditation or awareness can intercede in the process of creating this debris. It can discharge the energy around the event and can even discharge energy that has accumulated with past events.

Chapter 16

Meditation which began at unknown depths, and went on with increasing intensity and sweep, carved the brain into total silence, scooping out the depths of thought, uprooting feeling, emptying the brain of the known and its shadow. It was an operation and there was no operator, no surgeon; it was going on, as a surgeon operates for cancer cutting out every tissue which has been contaminated, lest the contamination should again spread.

—J. Krishnamurti

Meditation and Cosmic Debris Removal

As always there are many ways to accomplish any given task and so it is with cosmic debris removal. Many of these we can do ourselves while others require some help or facilitation from outside; this is the role of the healer. The discussion here will be limited to self-healing techniques. Facilitated healing will be discussed in the next section. However, there are a few basic principles that are fundamental to maintaining and cleansing our energy system.

The first principle is that there must be **movement**. That is movement in the energetic system, not mental or physical movement. *Cosmic debris* is essentially energy and information stored or locked away in our energy system.

The second principle is that for energy to flow it must form a **complete circuit**. In other words, it needs to have a ground, where the energy can go to be *recycled*.

Meditation

Meditation is one of the most difficult topics to write about. The experience of meditation is largely beyond description. No matter how much "experience" you have had with meditation there is always more to explore. Any given meditator may be just scratching the surface of meditation or may have explored the whole grand movement that is meditation. There is no way of knowing which, because the beauty of meditation is that it is not about measuring. It is a phenomenon without limits and without end. Thankfully there are no experts, therefore no one can invalidate your experience. A teacher will merely lead you to the door and once you pass through, it is your journey alone. In this context, any discussion of meditation is really an exploration.

With that in mind, let's explore meditation as an energetic phenomenon, not a deliberate act. The act of sitting and quieting the mind with various techniques may prepare one for meditation but it itself is not meditation. Preparing your mind and body is like opening a window—the breeze may or may not blow through the window. Meditation is the act of the breeze blowing in, not the opening of the window. Opening the window is partly achieved by removal of cosmic debris.

The word meditation comes from Sanskrit meaning to measure. What we have come to know as meditation starts when measurement is absent. The absence of measurement results in attention or awareness.

The beginning of meditation is to be aware of and stay with sensation (discomfort or pleasure) without labeling it. If we attend to an uncomfortable stuck spot in the body, then something will move—either your attention or the energy creating the sensation. If the attention moves away in thought, the energy will remain. If attention persists, the energy must move. In this way, cosmic debris can be cleared from our energy systems.

The state of no thought is not in itself meditation. Meditation is more than the absence of thought. A mind can be made empty, dull and thoughtless by smoking cigarettes and performing rituals. The quality of attention and understanding in the mind is all-important. The attentiveness has no relationship to the position the body is in. The body may be walking, sitting, lying down, driving a car it does not matter. It is only the choiceless quality of attention present that brings the meditative state and its accompanying release.

Meditation is the transmutation or transformation of energy. It will transform the cosmic debris associated with thought forms and thought form conglomerations and more.

Thought is a movement away from present time energy. Thought is escaping the *what is* associated with the event (emotional) that set up the energy formation. If one's attention stays with this stuck energy, without any movement away (thought), the energy form itself will have to move.

An inherent aspect of energy is nothing can stay the same over time. Entropy will soon see to its destruction. However, living organisms have the ability to hold entropy at bay to some extent. Meditation is an energetic phenomenon, it is not a deliberate act.

Meditation and the Aura

Humans have a way of storing experience in their energetic systems or auras. We even have information stored from other lifetimes. As the aura gets filled up with this information several things happen. Our energy system gets overloaded and our energy starts to stagnate from all the stuff held static in a dynamic field. The recording and storage of life experiences demands to be organized. Energy spent organizing and reorganizing this information prevents us from being in present time.

Leaving the door open for meditation means staying attentive to your aura and energy without any measurement (thought). Attending to these energetic packets of information transforms this energy, erasing the scars and clearing the field so innocence is regained. Understanding will be retained and the knowledge we use will continue to be available. Information that we forget, historical facts and figures, the knowledge of events, and technical data can be found in books, libraries and on the internet.

Information sticks when we resist. We resist because we are threatened or invalidated by the information. It is this resistance to invalidation that we are trying to make OK (usually through the process of becoming).

Meditation creates an unraveling process for these stuck out-of-time energies and information that are stored in the aura. Meditation will do more than clear the aura. As information is cleared, a revelation or insight may occur that leads to a greater understanding of oneself, the process of becoming and hence consciousness itself. This is the beginning of meditation; this is cosmic debris removal. This is healing.

Meditation at that hour was freedom and it was like entering into an unknown world of beauty and quietness; it was a world without image, symbol or word, without waves of memory. Love was the death of every minute and each death was the renewing of love. It was not attachment, it had no roots; it flowered without cause and it was a flame that burned away the borders, the carefully built fences of consciousness. It was beauty beyond thought and feeling; it was not put together on canvas, in words or in marble. Meditation was joy and with it came a benediction.

—J. Krishnamurti

Chapter 17

Cooperation comes into being only when there is love for the thing itself without the fear of punishment or failure, and without the hunger for success or recognition.

—J. Krishnamurti

Cooperation

Once we heal ourselves as individuals, then we can begin to heal ourselves as a group. All human beings on the planet are connected energetically, like one large organism. A healthy person in a sick society is like a healthy cell in a body that is dying of liver cancer. Waste products will eventually accumulate in the body and the individual cells won't get the nutrition they need. The whole body will suffer. When the body dies, all the cells die with it. What is the responsibility of the healthy individual to the rest of the organism or group?

Group healing occurs through cooperation instead of competition. Cooperation starts with the ability of a group to think together. Most twentieth-century cultures consider themselves civilized. Without the ability to think together, any culture is primitive no matter how grand the toys and gadgets.

To think together a group must be free of competition. The individuals in the group must have moved beyond the pettiness of competition. It needs to go deeper than just intellectually seeing the horrors of it. Not only must we be aware of the competitiveness in others but we must also see our own ruthless competition—from the most subtle to the outrageous. Only after competition has been thoroughly understood and no trace remains are we ready to think together and create in a cooperative fashion. This means you have no attachment to your opinions, you aren't compelled to defend them as if you were going to die. In your heart and soul as well as your head you have moved beyond competition and beyond fear.

To explore an issue without any attachment to one's own ideas is a truly beautiful phenomenon. The issue being explored can unfold in the group mind in a way that is not possible with the individual; it is a work of art, living poetry. Thinking together is the product of a group of mature human beings. It can only come about when you are secure enough in yourself that you need no external validation. You have nothing to prove to anyone, so there is no defensiveness.

Are you ready to do this? It is probably the hardest thing on earth, but also the most rewarding. It's rewarding not just for the information and understanding achieved but because it also fosters trust and love. These intangibles are necessary for community and group health, as no person is an island. Like all phenomena in this book, the intellectual communication of the subject does not do it justice. To be appreciated it has to be experienced.

To be healthy, we must speak of what we understand of truth. We must present what we see. In this there is no judgment, either externally in the group or internally, as to right or wrong. There is just presenting one's information, one's understanding with no attachment to it. This sharing of information is important because we are all unique and all have a different piece of the puzzle.

The defensiveness that arises when we are attached to an opinion interrupts the flow of energy and information in the group—the process will be blocked. There will be no thinking together, no cooperation. Again, how do we know if we are exploring truth or offering opinions? If you are unsure look into it, find out. Perhaps get a clairvoyant reading to help you see the difference.

Do we know the difference between pointing to truth and defending an opinion? How do you know truth when you see it? Is your truth different from my truth? There is a very popular movement in the last twenty years that insists that truth is different for each individual. It seems to grow out of the desire to avoid being judged for not knowing. The notion that your truth is different from someone else's because your experience is different is absolute immature nonsense.

Experience is not an approach to truth. There is not your truth based on your experience and my truth based on a different experience.

We all have different information from which we create our lives. These creations will work to varying degrees for each individual's purposes, but to call this information truth is silliness. There is only the wisdom derived from an intelligent understanding of the problem and a hypothesis as to a solution.

Positing a hypothesis or even a well-tested theory is never truth. There is truth in seeing a false process as a false process, such as the process of becoming more secure by imitating the ideal. This is inherent in any thought-based consciousness as thought always fragments the whole. When each individual in a group realizes this limitation, thought will be used as a tool to explore issues and options rather than as a cunning instrument to advance one's personal agenda. When a group thinking together understands this, cooperation will follow.

Section III

Facilitated Healing and Growth

Your health is in you and you do not observe it. Your ailment is from yourself and you do not register it.

—Sufi saying

Chapter 18

The cure of the part should not be attempted without the treatment of the whole. No attempt should be made to cure the body without the soul.
—Plato

Understanding the Modern Healer

The term healer is used here as we are beginning an era when many realize we need more than symptom relief from a health professional. A healer is one who embraces the whole person in context of the person's social and physical environment. When developing a treatment plan, a healer needs to consider the individual's life path and energetic cosmic influences.

A healer may practice a specific modality or use several modalities such as acupuncture, manipulation, bodywork, herbs, Qi Gong, aura healing, shiatsu or shamanism. The healer acknowledges, as foremost, the healing process and facilitates the individual's return to a sound state in body and mind as well as symptom relief. This is opposed to identifying with a particular modality that promises only symptom relief. A healer assists the individual in developing an understanding of the issues involved in the illness by providing the space for insight.

Some patients only want a "quick fix" treatment to address obvious symptoms. All people are not equipped to address the philosphical aspects of their illness. This may be part of an individual's life path and the healer needs to take this into account and not overtreat. Overtreating can invalidate the individual. Instead, a healer may prescribe a herbal remedy or medication to relieve the symptom and let the individual work on the underlying issues on his own. A healer may also provide some education along with the treatment.

Socially, we are coming to realize that the body is not a machine or a car. When the water pump breaks, replacing it does not fix the problem as it would in a car. When we are dealing with a body, the broken part or organ is just the symptom of a deeper problem. It is the healing of these deeper, more foundational issues that concerns the modern healer.

In its most dramatic form, this can be seen with organ transplant patients. A famous athlete recently had a cancerous liver replaced. Nonetheless, he died within a few months of the transplant. One could list all the biological reasons for the failure but underlying the biological reasons was the failure to correct unhealthy energy. Organ transplants would be more successful, and perhaps unnecessary, if the patient's unhealthy energy were dealt with prior to a transplant. If the issue is spiritual or emotional and it's accompanying *disturbed Qi* is not dealt with, the new organ may again malfunction.

To understand the modern healer we need to understand what it means to heal. According to Webster's dictionary *to heal* means to return to a sound state, whole. Also, it means to restore to original purity and integrity. This sounds a lot like getting in touch with our own oneness, to heal our relationship with ourselves, and ultimately God.

What does it really mean, to heal our relationship with ourselves? Is it the relationship between spirit and the body? What wounded the relationship to begin with? The nine steps to becoming whacko examined the role perfect pictures and invalidation play in becoming competitive and violent. From this we can see how the mental processes involved open the door to a whole host of unpleasant vibrations and emotions. When the body is full of unpleasant emotions such as fear and competition, spirit tends to leave. This opens the door wider for foreign energies to enter and the health of the individual deteriorates.

What prevents our healing? What prevents us from getting free of the process of becoming? Is it just habit or is it lack of understanding the mental processes? Do we like creating problems for ourselves? Do we like being violent and self-righteous and want to continue thinking we are immune from disease? Are we so fragmented we don't see the connection? Are we so caught up in the problem of the moment and illness appears so far away when we are healthy? What role does belief play in keeping us from the state of wholeness and integrity? Beliefs can create havoc with our energy system, creating stuck Qi that leads to tissue and organ dysfunction.

Beliefs are a step between thoughts and manifestation. Beliefs are the agents that enable us to form ethics from perfect pictures. They are essentially a thought that we are convinced is true. Beliefs are essentially frozen thoughts that are repeated over and over. The energy of a thought is somewhat ephemeral until it is given added weight. That added weight could come from the associated emotion the thought evoked, from reinforcement from an outside authority, or from our own strong-willed convictions.

Once we are convinced that our thought is true it has the effect of freezing or trapping the energy in our aura. This belief then begins to attract other energies to it (us). With these energies come people and events. It may be more correct to say these energies **are** people and events. This is how we create our life. It is through examining the manifestation that we grow and learn.

Some beliefs are bigger pitfalls than others. Some beliefs lead to clusters of beliefs and create a kind of block like a logjam on a river. They interfere with the flow of energy in the body or imbalance the energy system enough to lead to physical disease.

At this point it is important to understand that our beliefs are never truth, rather they are in conflict with truth. Beliefs will prevent understanding. Truth is always whole. Thoughts, and consequently beliefs, are always fragmentary. Understanding comes about through insight not through adopting a belief. One cannot build their way to truth with thought. Can you tell when you are operating from truth and insight rather than belief? How well do we know ourselves?

The role of the healer is to provide a fulcrum for change. A fulcrum is a point around which energy can reorganize itself.

Healers can facilitate reorganization by obviating the beliefs holding patients back. This should be done in a way that empowers, not invalidates, the patient. This is a very delicate dance for both healer and patient. Telling a patient that she is living a lie is rarely successful. To heal, patients must see lies for themselves. Healers can help by asking the right questions. A clairvoyant reading on the issue will usually work wonders. Once there has been an insight, the energy will be free to move. In this way the healer is a facilitator of growth.

Chapter 19

Faith and its lesser cousin belief are obstacles to understanding one's self.
They impede taking full advantage of the possibilities inherent in life.
—J. Krishnamurti

The Nuts and Bolts of Being
A Being of Light

Do we have a soul or spirit? As twenty-first century earthlings we are solidly steeped in a materialistic epistemology or worldview. This materialistic viewpoint makes acknowledging a spiritual component to our existence a difficult affair. Science has influenced public thinking a great deal in the twentieth century, undermining the credibility of organized religions and resulting in many people dismissing the notion of soul or spirit. While the churches may have had a warped idea of spirit and twisted it to benefit their own purposes, that is no reason to dismiss or ignore the concept entirely as science has done. Serious scientists, particularly subatomic physicists, are now acknowledging the influence of subtle energetic fields. Once again, many acknowledge some kind of spiritual aspect to themselves. This begs another question!

Are we a body with a spirit or spirit with a body? This is an important question if we are serious about our healing and growth. The answer is significant because it reflects who is senior in the relationship, who has control. Does the body outlast the spirit? Or does the spirit outlast the body? If so, does the spirit replace one body for another? Can spirit operate more than one body at the same time? How would that effect the energy available to this body?

As a result of clinical practice it has become clear that we are not a body with a spirit, we are a spirit with a body. Just as we in our bodies own cars and wear out one after another, we own bodies and wear them out one after another. This is a crucial concept if we are going to move toward understanding ourselves and taking responsibility for what we create. If we are body with a spirit, then the body and its intellect or thought makes rules and dictates action. This is how most of us operate currently. It is essentially the materialist view of the world, it is a product of thought and belief.

When thought finds its rightful place as a tool **guided by spirit,** then a new world unfolds. The right use of thought means there will be larger quiet spaces in the mind. Such spaces allow spirit's information to intimate itself upon the brain, hence finding expression. This is a necessary factor in good health.

Because we are spiritual beings we have the opportunity to forego the pettiness of the becoming process and create as spirit. Recognizing that spirit is senior to the body allows us take responsibility for what we are creating in our lives.

Spirit?

Already I hear people asking, "What is spirit?" Spirit is a quasi-energetic entity that exists within and/or without a body. Spirit has consciousness with or without being attached to a body. The reality that spirit experiences when in a body is more solid, much denser, and hence more vivid, with a sense of continuity. The reality that spirit experiences when not in a body is much like our own dream experiences. As a matter of fact, dreams are often out-of-body experiences. We create and take bodies for experience and growth.

Inherent in the concept of growth is the idea that one is more fully developed after the growth than before. As Albert Szent-Gyoergyi pointed out so eloquently in his paper, "There is a drive in living matter to perfect itself." What is this ultimate perfection? Is it always a drive toward perfection, and therefore a theoretical concept never realized in nature? Is it a reunion with the creator?

For everyday living, the drive toward perfection, not the realization of perfection, is most important. As we have seen in the section on disease and the divine purpose, the body through discomfort and illness, as well as joy, can point the way for development and change.

Auras

So we are energetic phenomena, beings of light. We are not energy or light in the usual sense of the word. The Chinese use the word Qi to describe this energy-like aspect of our being. Qi translates generally as life force. The term *kinesthetic medium* is perhaps more appropriate to describe the energy field surrounding us, as we can sense when somebody or something enters this field.

Morphic field is another term, used by Rupert Sheldrake. Morphic is used to reflect that the field may not be energy, strictly speaking, but a medium that contains information. Anyone interested in an intellectual and scientific debate about these fields may find Rupert Sheldrake's book, *The Presence of the Past: Morphic Resonance and the Habits of Nature* (Vintage 1988), satisfying.

This field or aura is very sensitive. For example, we can sense when somebody or something enters this field. Infants, even our pets have auras, and they can sense movement within their fields too. You and your pet can even sense movement in each other's field! We generate auras as spirit, but our spirit is more than our aura. Understanding our aura, however, helps us understand ourselves as spirit and the growth we experience as body and spirit.

This life force or subtle energy field is neither simple nor easily defined. Many people can see auras with the physical eye, while clairvoyants can see the layers and interpret the energy held within them. There are even instruments now available to practitioners that imitate the energy that emanates from the hands of healers who are practitioners of Qi Gong. In Qi Gong, the practitioner works with energy in ways that affects the body's energy channels and the aura.

The body, however, has its own very accurate instrument or gauge for detecting the quality and quantity of this life force—the radial pulse. Trained practitioners in oriental medicine read the pulse(s), which reveal in great detail the nature of the energy present. There are other indicators such as the spark in the eye, tongue, and pallor of the face and skin, or looking clairvoyantly. (More about the tool of looking clairvoyantly later.)

Since spirit can't be measured in inches and pounds, we must work with spirit, sensing and seeing its impact, as if we were studying its footprints. This is comparable to the way an electron microscope takes a picture by throwing electrons at an object and recording the electrons outlining the object. So too, we can look at where the body is as a reflection of the spirit that created it.

For example, is the body vibrant and expressive or is it robot-like and lifeless? A vibrant body often means a vibrant spirit, at home in the body. A body functioning like a robot doesn't necessarily mean that spirit is robotic. It more likely means that spirit isn't often in this body or isn't committing energetic resources to the body.

Many other indicators of spirit can be tracked. A person's lifestyle can often answer questions. What did spirit create for the body in this life? What is the person's occupation? How do they conduct themselves in relationship? This information provides a clear picture of the individual for the acupuncturist or clairvoyant.

Practitioners of energetic therapies or energetic medicine can go even further. Looking energetically or clairvoyantly at this ball of light we now know as spirit, we see or feel that it is not uniform. Clairvoyant looking provides a more intimate story of spirit and is usually done from a trance. The trance state does not mean the healer is unconscious, but is simply adjusting her energy in a particular way. This enables the clairvoyant to safely tune into the energies of another and look at them from a place of neutrality.

Most people do (and everybody can) feel each other's energy field either with their own energy field or their hands. There are different layers in this energy field also know as an aura. When looked at clairvoyantly, these layers have various qualities such as density, color or vibration, integrity, uniformity, etc. The layers are associated with the various energy centers or chakras that generate them. There are seven major internal body chakras and seven layers in the aura. There are many minor chakras that affect the major layers and patterns. However, if the major chakras are cleaned and balanced the minor chakras will generally take care of themselves.

Energetic classes will help you understand more about the aura, chakras and energy fields. These are experiential topics and should be explored more by everyone. Unfortunately, it is beyond the scope of this book to describe them in adequate detail. Take a class now!

Chapter 20

There is no illness of the body apart from the mind.
Socrates

Bioenergy System Basics

Understanding a few basic principles of bioenergy systems helps us understand how simple it is to get results with energy medicine. These principles apply to the animal world as well as the human body. You can even work with a plant's bioenergy system. And, bioenergy systems affect each other.

- *Energy in your space affects the energetic systems of those with whom you come in contact.*

Energy fields have fuzzy boundaries and interact with surrounding energy fields.

- *The quality of the field effects the quality and performance of every cell and tissue.*

The body is bathed in a subtle energy field. This field permeates every cell and every membrane.

- *A healthy energy field is a clean energy field.*

A mountain stream will support fish best if it is flowing and there is plenty of oxygen always renewing. If the stream slows and forms stagnant pools, unhealthy organisms move in and putrefaction results.

• Moving energy is essential for health. **Stagnation** creates disease.

Like a mountain stream, the energy field can only be clean if it is moving and cleansing itself.

• *Bioenergy systems are personal and unique, as this subtle energy is information.*

Bioenergy fields are not mechanical and impersonal like the electricity moving through the wires in your house. The kind of disease depends on the nature of the information and hence the layer of energy affected. The types and symptoms of the disease can range from acne to heart disease and fibromyalgia to depression.

•*Energy movement in a system requires a circuit, just like in the electrical system in a house. A circuit needs a source and a ground.*

In a house, the electrical system source is the power plant, and the electrical panel is wired to a copper rod in the ground. Sources for our bodies include the cosmos, the earth, or (hopefully your own) spirit. We ground to the earth or back up to spirit. Grounding recycles stagnant energy.

Chapter 21

*Be observant if you would have a pure heart, for something is born to you
in consequence of every action.*

—Jelaluddin Rumi

The Body Energies
The Cascade

Our bodies have several kinds of energy. Just as water cascades down
a mountain waterfall into a pool, over another drop into another pool,
and on down the mountain, so too our energy follows a similar cascade.
Starting with our energy as spirit, it moves into the body through the
chakras, out into our aura and into our etheric body. From the etheric
level, it bathes the body tissues and fills the meridians. This in turn
affects the energy at the biochemical level and determines the balance in
our physiology.

Illness and disease follow the same pathway or cascade. The cosmic
debris is generated by thought and cosmic influences and affects the
subtle energy fields of the **aura** and etheric bodies.

The Aura

The aura is a kinesthetic medium that surrounds the body and is
composed of the same kind of subtle energy as your thoughts. It contains
incredible amounts of information. It is kinesthetic, as the body can feel
when its aura bumps into something or someone. It transmits sensations
to your nerve endings. The quality of the energy in the aura affects the
other layers of energy in the body.

The aura itself is generated from your energy as spirit, earth energy,
cosmic energy, and energy and information generated by the body. The
aura flows within the body as well as around it. There are seven different

layers; each layer is associated with a different chakra. The strength of your aura is to a large degree determined by the strength and presence of you as spirit. If you are not in your body, your aura will be weak. Conversely, if you are very much in your body it will be stronger.

In this context the body's energy system is analogous to a lake storing the water at the top of a waterfall or cascade. You might think of the clouds that fill the lake as spirit, and the lake as your aura. The quality and quantity of the clouds and the precipitation they drop will determine the nature of the lake. The nature and quantity of water in this lake affect everything downstream: the waterfall, the river below the waterfall and the people in the town who will use and drink the water. If we think of the cascading waterfall and the river that carries water to the towns and people as the energy in the meridian system carrying the energy to the cells and organs, we have an analogous model for the human energy system.

Meridan Level

The **meridian level** is a network of channels or pathways in the body along which Qi energy flows. There are many points along these channels where decreased electrical resistance can be found. These points are also known as acupuncture points. Different points have different purposes and different qualities. Some points will increase the flow of energy into a meridian while others will decrease the flow and may direct it to another meridian. This is similar to sluice gates in an irrigation system.

Energy can be summoned or coaxed to flow through channels by various means of stimulation such as holding or pressing a point, inserting a needle, burning moxa on or over the point, laser light stimulation, magnets, vibrations from tuning forks, etc. The primary principle of a healthy energy system at this level is balance as well as flow. The body needs a **balance** of flow in all meridians, and from right to left sides in the given meridians. An imbalance will set up a situation of **excess** or **deficiency**.

If we continue with our mountain stream analogy, let's assume that there are many different communities fed by the water from the lake. Many different streams are needed to deliver the water to each community. If a stream channel becomes blocked by debris from fallen logs, there will be a community downstream that will run out of water and its inhabitants will eventually die of thirst. Conversely, if an irrigation gate is left open, one community will flood while another thirsts. Since the blood and nutrient flow to the cells are determined by Qi flow, balance is crucial.

Each meridian in the body feeds a community of cells. If they don't receive their Qi, they won't receive their nutrients and the information needed for healthy functioning. They will starve for nutrients, drown in their own garbage, or malfunction due to the wrong information. Illness will result. Likewise, if a mountain stream is being fouled by a herd of elk with *girardia* then the water delivered to the community will be fouled and the inhabitants will become ill.

So too, every cell in the body needs to be supplied with fresh healthy Qi to thrive in a healthy manner. Hydraulic engineers will balance or regulate the flow of water to communities by opening and closing dams and sluice gates. Acupuncturists work in similar fashion opening and regulating acupuncture points to balance the flow in the meridians.

We find deficiency/excess phenomena at all levels of the cascade or energy system. The clouds (spirit) may not provide enough rain for the lake to feed the streams. In body terms, this means a deficiency in etheric vitality and a weak aura. The lake water itself may be deficient in oxygen or the water molecules may have too much of an unhealthy isotope of hydrogen, or too much algae and silt. A lake without enough oxygen or a proper balance of nutrients will cause a host of problems for the biologic life living in the lake. Similarly our body will suffer from a host of problems if it doesn't have the proper balance of clean healthy energy or Qi.

Etheric Level

The etheric level is analogous to ground water, to continue our hydrologic example. It provides a storage reservoir for important core energies that are necessary for maintaining the body. The etheric body can become contaminated with toxic energy just as toxins seep down into the ground water.

Depletion in the etheric body has direct consequences on the health of the physical body. Just as a town's well may dry up in a drought, the etheric level can be drained if not replenished. The etheric body is made of different core energies and vibrations that have to be present in order to keep the physical body healthy.

The **etheric level** (also known as the etheric template or etheric double) provides the template or energetic structure for the physical body. A deficiency of etheric vitality can result in fatigue and depression. Physical as well as emotional traumas will affect this laye. Freeing these chinks in the template relieves most aches and pains, especially back pain. To work on this level, a practitioner should apply slight pressure to the body or bones until he feels a wavelike sensation. Follow or ride the wave to set the issue free.

Biochemical Level

The **biochemical** layer is the last to be effected and the one we are most familiar with due to its exposure in the media. The subtle energy layers influence meridian level energies which in turn have a direct effect upon the tissues and glands. This can be positive if the energy is healthy. If the energy is unhealthy or out of balance, it can create aberrant physiology or biochemistry. The energy field can stimulate or regulate the glands such as the pituitary to secrete normal or abnormal amounts of hormones. This can easily start a chain reaction of biochemical events in the body.

The Influences

Our energy field is influenced both from forces around us and within ourselves. Most illness is created by a combination of effects at all layers of the energy system.

Everything in our lives has a vibration or reflects and absorbs vibration. For example, the influence of the heavenly bodies affects all and is felt by many. These influences can be charted through astrological studies. The earth's energy, which varies greatly with geographical location, also affects us. The influence of architecture, with its ability to reflect, affect, transform and deform energy is greatly undervalued and underestimated in western culture. And, most importantly, the energy of other people impacts the energy in our environment and frequently the energy within our own space.

The strength, health and makeup of our own energy system

determine our susceptibility to outside energies. Sensitive constitutions are more greatly effected than dense constitutions. Factors influencing sensitivity include planetary influences at birth, a weak aura, and neglect of the body. If we are sensitive, we will most likely feel everything and everybody. This does not mean that the sensitive person is less healthy or that her aura will suffer more damage than the dense person. However, she will feel every little disturbance. This sensitivity enables her to get out of harms way before the damage is done.

We commonly trigger a disturbance in our aura when we annoy someone. If he projects his annoyance with you via his energy field, your energy field reacts with a headache, stomachache or that old familiar feeling "there's a knife in my back." If the person is a casual acquaintance and you quickly leave the area, he willl forget about you and the discomfort will disappear. If you annoy someone you live with day after day, it can create more problems. If it continues for months and years, it will progress from a nonspecific malaise or set of symptoms to a more classically defined illness.

If the person you offended retaliates and projects energy at your third chakra (solar plexus), you may experience a stomach ache and digestive difficulties. Third chakra disturbances impact the stomach, pancreas, gallbladder and liver. This energy could create a hyperactivity of the digestive system and an excess or deficiency of acid. Each person and each situation is unique. Taking digestive aids whether pharmaceutical derivatives or herbals will be merely palliative. The energy will remain and continue to do its damage. The drug, may clear the symptoms but the energy will have gone deeper and is causing deterioration in one of the organs. It may not be noticed for days, weeks or months until a more serious problem shows itself, such as an ulcer or worse.

The beliefs, pictures and thoughts present in our auras largely determine our susceptibility to energetic invasions. Foreign energy resonating with our own pictures will stick to us. Without resonance, there is nothing for the energy to stick to and there will be no invasion. Love and compassion are the vibrations we like to have in our space. When we radiate love and compassion internally, we can expect love and compassion to be drawn to us.

Psychic Attacks

We are likely to assault another's energy when we fail to express our feelings. If Bob's angry and afraid to tell Lucy, then Bob will probably invade Lucy's space. Bob's anger will fill his aura and spill over into Lucy's space and aura. She immediately will feel uncomfortable and sense something is wrong. Lucy does not have to be in the same room or even in the same building. If Bob expresses his anger verbally, much energy is released and Lucy will suffer much less. If Bob tries to keep it inside, more energy gets directed at Lucy's subtle energy levels and the attack is more virulent and insidious.

Psychic attacks create stagnation in the aura and the meridians, particularly affecting the Liver and Gallbladder channels. This stagnation over time will develop into an excess condition and create heat in the body. The heat will then rise to the head, intensifying the headache already present from having someone in your space. In addition to the stomachache and headache, we may end up with itchy eyes, rash on the face, and a hard wiry pulse. The symptoms can be many and varied depending on personal histories and how long the energy has been present. The variables are too numerous to list.

Healing the Disturbances

An acupuncturist would treat a psychic attack at the meridian level, tonifying the weakened Qi in the body. Strengthening the Qi in the body may enable the individual to push out the invader's Qi. The success of tonification alone would depend on the relative strengths of the energies involved. If tonification, is insufficient, then any evil Qi still in the meridian should be removed. If the offending party is no longer in the area or in the aura, that would be the end of it.

If the angry person's energy still lingers in the aura, she may experience the invasion again shortly after she leaves the office. The psychic healer would look at the patient's aura, to clear the offending energy, and look at the issues that attracted the situation in the first place. The stagnation would linger in the Liver channel but probably clear within a day or two. The most effective treatment, leaving the least chance of recurring symptoms, would be a combination of clearing both the subtle energy field and the meridian level.

Chapter 22

Fame has also this great drawback, that if we pursue it we must direct our lives in such a way as to please the fancy of men, avoiding what they dislike and seeking what is pleasing to them.

—Benedict Spinoza

Is Medical Science Making Us Sick?

An article in the Colorado Springs Gazette (October 3, 1999) stated, "Lucian Leape, a Harvard University professor who conducted the most comprehensive study of medical errors in the United States, has estimated 1 million patients nationwide are injured by errors during hospital treatment each year and that 120,000 die as a result. Their 1991 report found that one of every 200 patients admitted to a hospital died as a result of a hospital error." These numbers roughly represent the 5-10 percent of errors that actually get reported. "It's by far the No. 1 problem" in health care said Leape, an adjunct Professor of health policy at the Harvard School of Public Health.

The Colorado Springs Gazette (October 4, 1999) reports the findings of Robert Helmreich, a professor of psychology at the University of Texas at Austin, who spent two decades studying the behavior of aviation and aerospace crews as well as medical settings. In surveys, he has found pilots and doctors hold markedly different attitudes about their capabilities. Roughly 60 percent of surgeons and anesthesiologists responded they perform effectively when fatigued, compared with 30 percent of pilots. "They deny overwhelmingly the influence of fatigue," Helmreich said. "There's a certain climate in which the surgeon can say, 'I'm the surgeon and I'm infallible'. The perfectionism that drives many in medicine also can render them vulnerable to overconfidence that escalates into arrogance and reinforces competitiveness."

Although the above newspaper articles paint dark pictures of

119

modern medicine, the damage done by institutionalized medicine is more common and subtle than the article illustrates. Even if these medical errors never happened, a sensitive investigator would still have to answer the yes to the question: Is medical science making us sick? This book is concerned less with the blatant errors than it is with the apparent victories and successes. Of course, no nurse or doctor wants to hurt any patient. No doctor wants to make patients sicker or have to come back for more treatment. The healer is faced with the unfortunate truth that most drug cures are hollow victories.

Eradicating the symptoms of disease with drug treatments compromises the patient's energy system, setting the stage for disease later on. This may be acceptable if there were no other way to treat illness. However, many medical practitioners now know alternatives to traditional drug-oriented medicine. Alternative therapies involve less risk to the patient and greater likelihood of long term success. Most importantly, they offer the patient spiritual and physical opportunities for growth.

Becoming acquainted with the Chinese Materia Medica was a humbling experience for me. Over a thousand years ago, Chinese doctors documented the effects of hundreds of herbs in much greater detail and completeness than pharmacists document the drugs of today.

Chinese physicians understood the effect each herb had on the body. They knew the specific meridians it entered, the direction of the effect, whether it would it would make the body hotter or colder and other important qualities. They would combine different herbs to achieve the particular effect they wanted to restore health and balance as well as treating the symptom.

Modern science does not concern itself with overall balance within the body's energy system but rather with just the treatment of the symptom. This satisfies the general public, who want to be free of symptoms as soon as possible. A look at the nature of science and the history of modern medicine helps put the issue in perspective.

Anyone serious about life, has inevitably turned a skeptical eye towards our medical system. The modern healthcare system is a very complex web of high powered marketing with top dollar advertising, new miracle drug discoveries, high tech surgery, lucrative research grants and many sick people. It represents an amazing amount of manpower and money headed in a particular direction with a great degree of certainty and momentum.

The foundations of medical science are rarely questioned, except in the circle of modern healers. Such healers treat a stream of patients addicted to prescription medications and surgeries that in many cases leave them in worse shape than when they started. Medications often produce a long list of unpleasant symptoms, called *side effects* by the drug manufacturers' marketing personnel.

Ironically, most of these patients aren't even aware that the medication or surgery is responsible for their current complaint. A spade, whether you call it a shovel or a digging implement, is still a spade. The effects of a drug include all effects not just the aspect that removes symptoms. If a drug treats heartburn and destroys your liver and kidneys, one could easily say the drug destroys liver and kidneys and incidentally it removes the symptom of heartburn from the body. The term "side effect" is strictly a marketing tool. A clue nonetheless as to the motivations behind the drug-based medical approach.

The Nature of Science

The nature of science revolves around the study of cause and effect. The most it can do is provide a description of phenomena. The description may be just of an effect or it may include a theoretical explanation of cause. This explanation is essentially a description of a mechanism whereby cause creates effect.

Science can never prove a description or any theory to be true. It can only prove a description or mechanism to be a false explanation. The description can be verbal or mathematical, but the description is never the thing described. Truth is always outside of the proof. The description may assign statistical probabilities to a phenomenon based on test results enabling one to make predictions. So where is the rub?

In order to conduct rigorous scientific research, scientists must be able to identify and isolate the variables involved. In order to design and accurate experiment scientists must be able to isolate a sample within which all relevant variables are controlled. The discussion then must center on what is a relevant variable.

Western medical research has focused on cause and effect within a biochemical model. The model assumes aberrant biochemistry is the cause or basis of disease and organ dysfunction. Even in the case of invading organisms the method of action is through biochemical processes. The assumption is that if we correct the biochemical imbalance we cure the disease. Basing research on the biochemical model of disease also enables scientists to design studies based on what appears to be a closed system. The studies have the appearance of being able to establish control groups that are uniform with respect to the relevant variables.

This requires a **belief** that an invisible force does not regulate biochemistry. The rsearcher then must believe that spiritual subtle energy and the Qi of oriental medicine do not exist or at least affect the biochemistry of the body in any way. However, at this time there are results to the contrary.

Nonetheless, the momentum of the present system keeps pushing more and more drug treatments. Prescription drug therapy is at an all time high. The most commonly prescribed group of medications are the antidepressants. These drug treatments have very serious side effects. This is particularly depressing because most emotional disorders are readily treated with energetic therapies.

It is an obvious fact to energetic practitioners that biochemistry is indeed influenced and controlled by subtle energetic forces. It is also a fact that every person's energy system is unique, thereby negating the ability of scientific researchers to control relevant variables. This makes it impossible to create an accurate control group. Thus, medical science is not a strict science it is rather pseudoscience. This is not to say that many useful discoveries and inventions don't result from the pseudoscience of medical research. However, one needs to be very careful as to the authority we ascribe to its products.

In summary, science cannot treat the whole person. Experiments cannot be designed to take into account the whole person. Scientific experiments by their very nature are fragmentary. It is becoming popular for some medical doctors to use acupuncture to treat specific symptoms. These treatments will not be treating the whole person and will most likely create imbalance in the process of removing the symptom. While it is far preferable to drug therapy, the patient is being shortchanged. If it is a medical treatment proven by science to be effective, we can be sure it doesn't treat the whole person.

Chapter 23

Great minds have always encountered opposition from the mediocre.
—Albert Einstein

Science as Authority

If medical science is fragmentary and does not treat the whole person, why is it so popular? Why does it have such authority? Is it that discoveries of new surgical techniques and new drugs make great sound bites? Is it the marketing? Is it the medical association's political lobby? Is it because it works? It is all of these and perhaps none of these. It may be that when we are in pain and don't know what is the cause and effect, we are very susceptible to giving up our power to an authority that claims to have a treatment.

Many alternative practitioners follow the same path as the M.D. Treat the symptom with a short office visit, prescribe expensive supplements and come back next week so the expert doctor can continue fixing you. In contrast the goal of the modern healer is self-healing. To empower the patient with the tools and information to understand the issue and clear the energy behind the illness.

Society assumes that doctors have successful treatments. The modern medical industry with its high tech treatments and constantly changing pharmacy make it very difficult for the patient to understand and take responsibility for his course of therapy. The intimidation from the language and medical equipment demand we turn over our power. This loss of control over our health and body invites vibrations of futility, helplessness and victimization. These energies contribute to our illness or start creating a new one.

Aside from the intimidation of the medical profession there is a tendency in all of us, when we are over our heads, to rely on outside authorities. When a patient walks or is carried in the door with some painful debilitating disease, most medical professionals initially feel they are in over their heads. As practitioners, we have all asked ourselves: "What in the world can I do for this person?" It would be convenient to rely on an outside authority's prescribed treatment. Who wants the responsibility? Scientific research provides us with that outside authority, an authority that will usually hold up in court and absolve us of responsibility and feelings of inadequacy when a treatment falls short of the mark.

Science is the ideal tool (even scapegoat) for the corporation that turns medicine into a for profit business. The doctor becomes a technician, an intermediary, between the patient and researcher. The doctor examines patients and orders tests. Based on the results (the aberrant biochemistry), the doctor prescribes the drug deemed appropriate by the research. The divine purpose of the disease is lost, usually not even given a fleeting thought.

The doctor, in order to treat, is totally dependent on the research and information of someone else. With so much contradictory research on any given topic, the official line changes frequently in many areas of medicine. After more than 15 years of research, scientists still disagree on the causative factors for AIDS. The medical community was once adamant that HIV was the infectious agent. New research in the late 1990s is proving that to be a false conclusion. Not knowing the cause has not stopped the presciption of very expensive and toxic drug treatments.

Whose research is our doctor using—a graduate student at a university or major drug company? This should give any prospective patient pause. In the seventies, the author was infected with *girardia lamblia* an intestinal parasite found in streams. After several months of intestinal difficulties and nearly loosing consciousness from dehydration, he finally relented and visited an M.D. The initial M.D. suspected girardia and ordered tests saying he would prescribe metronidazole if the test were positive. The original M.D. went on vacation and the stand-in prescribed quinacrine hydrochloride instead. He felt it was less toxic, and that metronidazole was carcinogenic. Who do you believe? Did they get their information from different drug companies? Did they read different research?

Twenty years later the author again encountered girardia from drinking contaminated water. This time acupuncture was widely available. An acupuncture treatment and a clairvoyant reading brought about full recovery.

In his book, *Working in the Void*, Michael Greenwood, M.D., sums up the situation poetically:

I was trained in a model of single diagnosis and the treatment of symptoms, which I now know misses the point. Anything we put in our mouths with the aim of eradicating symptoms misses the point. It matters not whether it is a drug, an herb or a homeopathic remedy. Our intention is all-important. If the intention is to eradicate symptoms, symptoms may be eradicated, but in the long run, healing may be deferred.

With oriental medicine and other energetic treatments, causative factors and mechanisms of causation are not necessary for treatment. Just assessing the imbalance or energy deficiency and bringing it back into balance will allow the body to heal itself.

Chapter 24

Much madness is divinest sense—
To discerning eye—
Much sense—the starkest Madness
                    —Emily Dickinson

Science has become a Political Issue

Even though medical science is not a true science that doesn't mean that it's invalid. Many inventions and discoveries have come about through *pseudoscience*. Much of the confusion arises when organizations such as the American Medical Association and Food and Drug Administration regularly approve procedures based on pseudoscientific research or tradition. Other procedures are outlawed because they were proven effective not through hard scientific research but rather by "junk science." Approval has changed from a medical or scientific basis to a political tool, used to withhold insurance payments and direct the media and public towards certain types of treatments.

Some alternative treatments are supported by thousands of years of experience but ignored by mainstream physicians and denigrated by drug manufacturers. Meanwhile a popular antidepressant drug with only a few years of research and a list of thirty side affects can be dispensed like candy, often to toddlers and infants. In many cases the companies that profit from the sales conduct the actual research on these drugs. The same companies also provide doctors with information on drug usage and dosage. These same companies hire lobbyists to influence legislators to create legislation that will make it easier for them to do what they do—sell drugs. In some instances legislators are simultaneously making it more difficult for alternative methods of treatment that require no drugs or operations.

As mentioned earlier in Section I - Illness and the Divine Purpose, overriding a disturbed energy system with techno-biomedical devices and drugs can actually hinder the purpose that we are actually here to achieve. In addition to missing the opportunity for growth, most drug-based treatments have serious side effects; one need only to consult a nurse's drug guide to see how serious this really is. Even if the person taking the drug does not experience the classic side effect to a debilitating degree, the drug still wreaks havoc in his system. Yes, medical science really is making us sick—not just individually with drugs but as a society with the politicking and media hype around their products. Some drugs can be lifesaving. However, fostering the idea that taking drugs is the solution to simply feeling out of sorts diminishes the divine in all of us.

On the other hand, in emergency and critical conditions it can actually buy a person time to get the rest of her healing in order. In the case of an athlete, whose purpose is to experience what it is like to be a world class or world famous athlete, biomedical intervention may make the goal possible. But at what cost to the body, maybe none or maybe at great expense, depending on the individual situation. In many instances a more holistic therapy may have achieved the same ends with less costly consequences. There are no hard and fast rules that work for everyone and every situation. In the end we must rely on our own resources, intuition, clairvoyance, and intelligence to guide us in achieving the creation that feeds our ultimate spiritual healing.

Chapter 25

Never ignore those intuitions. When you feel a slight repugnance to doing
something, listen to it. These premonitions come from God.
                                    —Jelaluddin Rumi

Choosing the Right Modality for You

As health care practitioners, people come to us with pain and
illness, they want their symptoms to go away. Patients don't usually come
for a treatment and ask to find the reason for their pain so they can heal
themselves. They very rarely come to an appointment for a treatment or
reading so they can stay healthy. Instead, they ask: can you treat back
pain? Can you treat migraines, epilepsy, diabetes, colitis, etc?

If you don't make the symptom disappear or dramatically improve in
a couple of sessions, then you may be seen as a charlatan or just plain
incompetent. It then becomes a dance of education, of how and when to
let them get a glimpse of the cause. What are the issues that set up this
energetic, now physical malady? If you broach the subject before you
have their trust, they will not be back. If you wait too long, the symptom
will be gone, not the issue, and they won't be back.

There are as many different ways to do this dance of facilitating
another's healing as there are healers. With so many new schools of
alternative healing styles and techniques being developed every year how
is one to know what do and when? Who do you believe and how do you
know when someone is incompetent?

The best answer is the simplest one, use your clairvoyance. I can
hear the objections already, people believing they are not clairvoyant.
We are all clairvoyant to one degree or another we have just learned not
to trust our pictures. When a friend or acquaintance offers a referral, do
you get an inkling of whether you would like to check it out or not? Is

the inkling an instinctive feeling or is it prejudice spun out by the intellect?

That inkling is information coming to you through your sixth chakra, your energy and information center responsible for clear seeing. Do you just accept the advice of your friend and go because you trust them? Do you trust your friend more than you trust yourself? This is giving away your power, but usually much more helpful than picking the largest ads in the yellow pages. Do you get several referrals from friends and then call the practitioners to get a sense of who you are most comfortable with? Then do you listen and trust this feeling or is it overruled by rationalizations, such as, well Bob or Betty liked him so he must be good or she went to Harvard and has five degrees.

Do you not get the help you need or would like because you want to save the money for a new car or refrigerator? Do you wait until you are flat on your back before you seek assistance? Any practitioner may be *good*, but good for whom is the critical part. There are some basic questions we can ask ourselves to narrow our search.

To Drug or Not to Drug?

Biochemical-based drug therapies circumvent the purpose for which we created the disease in the first place. This is not surprising—in the western medical mind there is no purpose to disease, it is something to be rid of. Western drug-based therapies have a place in critical care, especially in auto accidents, heart attacks, terminal illness and the like. The greater the deterioration in the body or the more life-threatening the disease, the more appropriate a drug or surgery-based treatment.

1.) Is the illness or injury clearly and imminently life threatening? Will the individual bleed to death before morning, or will the wound heal properly without stitches, are they conscious, are they breathing, are there possibly broken bones, are there possible internal injuries with internal bleeding, blood in stools, lumps, chest pain with profuse sweating? This list is by no means all-inclusive.

These indications all obviously require attention by a competent western trained M.D., before seeking out energetic treatments and alternative or complementary therapies.

2.) Is the disease more of a nuisance than a threat to life?
Problems include: soft tissue injuries, back pain, sprains and strains, digestive problems, minor allergies, asthma, mild or moderate fevers, aches and pains, fatigue, anxiety, immune system disorders, rashes, insomnia, and depression.

These symptoms can be appropriately treated by energetic or non-drug alternative therapy. As in all things, common sense must be used. If one is prone to severe asthma attacks you don't throw your inhaler away the first month because acupuncture has been helping.

3.) Is the illness a nuisance with the potential of it becoming life threatening?
This includes illnesses such as diabetes, asthma, lupus, some allergies. It may be prudent to use both drug or surgery treatments in conjuction with energetic treatments.

Dermatological and some minor surgeries such as skin cancers can be an appropriate use of medical technology. Even though a weakness in one's Qi that keeps skin healthy may be the underlying cause of the cancer, a simple superficial surgery can save the life of the patient. If the patient is 60+ years old, they could have been abusing their Qi and exposing themselves to harsh UV rays for most of that time. In this case it could take many years to rebuild the energy system to the point that it would heal the cancerous lesion. The patient would likely die before healing would occur. Knowing what battles to fight and on what levels is a personal decision that is best made with an understanding of the whole person, especially their energy system. There will always be situations where the appropriate modality for the job is not a clear choice.

40-year-old male. Generally excellent health. Presenting with 18 fatty lesions or lumps just under the skin ranging in size from half an inch to one-and-a-half inches in diameter. The first one appeared about 20 years previously. Physical and emotional abuse in childhood, lost his father to a prolonged illness in early teenage years. Some lumps were painful especially in areas where contact was unavoidable during activities such as sleep and yoga. A clairvoyant reading revealed that he had walled off pockets of pain from these earlier experiences. He had done extensive healing around these issues but the lumps remained. He made a few attempts to reduce them with acupuncture and other energetic means but they remained. Eventually he explored surgery as they were very superficial and a cosmetic surgeon assured him there would be virtually no scars. The incisions were no more than half an inch for the largest lesion. He had always experienced tightness in the area between abdomen and chest. Rolfing and yoga eased it some but essentially it remained. He had difficulty standing erect and breathing deeply. When a lesion at the bottom of the sternum was removed the relief was immediate. His chest expanded and he breathed easier. He reported a sense of well-being as soon as the restricted energy was released. Some of the lumps returned a week later in approximately the same areas. They were again removed. This time they returned in different areas and some were once again removed. The torso remained more open and free but still contained a good deal of restriction. Some lumps returned but not all. Apparently he is not able or ready to experience and release the painful feelings which for the most part revolved around the issue of rejection.

How Do You Select between Alternative Therapies?

All illness is inherently spiritual. It all starts at the subtle energy level and cascades downward until finally reaching the physical tissues of the body. Any therapist should be fully versed in energetic medicine since as spirit we are, first and foremost, energy. An energetic component is our most basic level, the root of the disease.

Preferably, the practitioner will be thoroughly trained in a *whole system approach*. The best example of this is oriental medicine. With oriental medicine one can determine how any substance or even a change of climate will affect the body. The practitioner can determine how all herbs, drugs, foods, beverages will affect the overall balance of an individual's constitution. The practitioner will know whether these items will aggravate the disease factors or if it will promote health. The conscientious health care provider will want to promote health and not just treat the symptom. More of this will be discussed later under the section on oriental medicine.

A basic guide in selecting treatment is how long has the patient had the disease and is it life threatening? Below are some questions to use as a basic triage. Keep in mind that every individual is unique. It requires a personal judgment call to intervene in an illness on the energetic level or a biochemical level. The least invasive treatment, with the fewest side effects, will be an energetic intervention, lifestyle and/or dietary changes.

A brief list of these treatments is in order. I would approach them for myself, starting at the purely spiritual energetic levels. Self-healing techniques/classes, clairvoyant reading, aura healing, Natural Force Healing, and Qi Gong. If little or no change occurs, then move to a more physical level energetic treatment such as Acupuncture, Zero Balancing, Vector Therapy or core (etheric level) integration, cranial sacral therapy, or shiatsu. If little or no response occurs at this point, then it would be prudent to move to a more physical level of treatment such as massage, rolfing, soma, naturopathic manipulation, chiropractic adjustments, or hydrotherapy (hot/cold contrast therapy).

Depending on the specific nature of the problem, herbal and homeopathic treatments can be added to the physical level of treatment. It is important not to abandon the energetic level work during the more physical level therapies. The most lasting and rapid change happens when work takes place on more than one level. Even if no real illness is present, it is important for health maintenance to address both the physical and energetic levels such as getting bodywork, doing yoga or tai chi, and spiritual level work such as clairvoyant reading classes.

If the disease has a long history and much tissue has already been damaged, then more physical level treatments may be necessary for change. It may be heart disease, liver or kidney damage and, if it is life threatening, life saving drug treatments or surgery may be necessary. If the heart's blood vessels are blocked, surgery may be the only way to create change rapidly enough to keep the heart beating.

There is a point when the organ or body is so deteriorated that there is little sense in trying to repair it. Let the tissue return to the earth from which it came. From an eternal spirit standpoint, it is a simple matter— you drop one body, take another and start the process all over again. However, for the body this is all too permanent because the body doesn't get another chance and is very frightened.

How much of society's resources should we direct to saving people who have thoughtlessly trashed their bodies? This is a difficult question for society to answer. How much should society invest in someone who has lived an abusive life, polluting the body by smoking cigarettes, eating a high fat diet overloaded with sweets, no exercise, to basically give them another year, or several years? Some operations cost well into the six figures, demanding insurance money from us all. Is it worth it? How much money is another year of life worth in dollars? It is one thing if it is covered by the individual's savings and another if it is an expense for the insurance companies. If that extra year is spent in poor health or in pain, then what is the value?

Below are some basic questions to help sort out where to go for help and when:

1.) How long has the disease been in the body? Is it a chronic, long-term degenerative disease such as arthritis?

If the disease has been in the body a long period of time and has progressed to a chronic condition, then herbal or biochemical interventions, in other words a more physical level treatment as well as an energetic treatment would be most effective.

2.) Is the disease or symptom less than three months old? Is it back pain, aches, pains, digestive upsets, depression, insomnia, headaches, anxiety attacks, or fatigue?

Illness of recent onset is still mostly in the energetic not the physical realm, and will quickly respond to energetic treatment. In a small percentage of cases there is a slight danger because some illnesses are present in the body for a long period of time, unknown to the individual. Such diseases exhibit innocuous symptoms such as fatigue in the case of a slowly growing cancer.

With this in mind, it never hurts to get a diagnosis from a western medical doctor and then weigh your options for treatment with a practitioner of whole systems healing. However, if you are diagnosed with a non-life threatening disease and you choose to take a drug treatment without pursuing any energetic methods first, you very well may be hurting yourself.

3.) Are the symptoms less than three years old?

If so, this is still a relatively fresh manifestation and should respond very well to energetic treatments. Food and environmental sensitivities, digestive upsets, heartburn, aches pains, headaches, moodiness are typical symptoms.

If someone has had the disease more than six months, it may not be acutely life threatening. More esoteric and energetic means of treatment should be considered. Again, choose energetic modalities first because they address the illness/issue at a more core or foundational level as opposed to treating symptoms. Responsible energetic healing promotes health, and has no toxic side effects. It actually feels relaxing and even euphoric, a natural high if you will. When we are healthy and our energy flows freely, a pleasant euphoric state is the common experience.

The longer the symptom or illness has been in the body, the longer it takes to return the system to energetic health and balance with energetic interventions. If an illness has taken several years, say twelve, to go from the subtle spiritual energetic levels to the physical, that energetic pattern is not going to be turned around in three treatments. Expect to work on the issue for many months or even several years.

A reading or acupuncture treatment is not to be confused with the instant responses of antibiotic types of drugs. On some occasions an energetic treatment can get results even more quickly than the most powerful drugs. The common cold or flu is a good example. The cold virus energetic vibration can be erased psychically and within seconds cold symptoms will virtually disappear.

4.) Are you basically healthy and want to stay that way?

This is the time to explore the health maintenance tools and options available to you. Explore different treatments and health care practitioners. Develop a relationship with several health care providers so when you are in a crisis you know where you can go for help. Incorporate healthy activities into your life on a daily basis.

The negative effects from drinking lots of coffee and smoking cigarettes on a daily basis for twenty years are obvious. Instead of burdening the body, do a little health promotion every day. Then, we will have made an enormous impact over twenty years. we can't go wrong with twenty minutes of yoga or tai chi and a glass of vegetable juice instead of coffee. Eating high performance foods for a high performance organism (your body), only makes sense as does receiving energy and the bodywork of your choice.

There are so many different types of energy work and most will be of some benefit. As a general guideline, who the practitioner is as a person is more important than what system they use. Obviously the sensitive and intelligent healer will select sensitive and intelligent modalities to employ. Bodywork is largely the same story; it varies tremendously from practitioner to practitioner even among those using the same system.

Bodywork systems that organize the structure of the body such as rolfing, soma, and those systems modeled on Ida Rolf's approach, incorporate a bit of wisdom that sets them apart. This wisdom is put into practice by releasing stuck tissues in a way that aligns the body around a vertical axis. Realignment has the effect of promoting smoother energy flows throughout the body. Some bodyworkers work largely energetically even though they use a physical modality. Others have an entirely physical approach. It is really up to you to find something that works for you. The differences can be subtle or vast. The only way is to sample a few or use your clairvoyance to find what you need.

Energy work that operates on the subtle levels is important to include in maintenance regimes for optimizing health. Modalities such as aura healings, Natural Force Healing, Zero Balancing, clairvoyant readings will not only remove cosmic debris and balance our energy system but will assist us in getting in touch with our life goals. To really take charge of your life and healing process, seek out Self-Healing classes that teach you how to run energy through your energy system as well as many psychic self-healing techniques. If you are basically healthy and need a little fine-tuning, Five Element acupuncture can do wonders to rebalance your energy system and help your body adjust to the change of seasons.

Chapter 26

Discontent is the want of self reliance—it is infirmity of will.
                                        —Ralph Waldo Emerson

Stick Me, Pound Me, Bake Me, Plug Me Into the Wall Baby!

Oriental Medicine (Stick Me)

Oriental medicine is probably the best example we have on the planet of a whole system's approach to health and healing. Oriental medicine considers all aspects of a person: physical, mental/emotional, spiritual, energetic, and biochemical. It does so from a perspective of balance between the five phases (earth, metal, water, wood, and fire) and the principles of Yin/Yang theory. This can be further delineated into eight principles (yin/ yang, hot/cold, internal/external, and excess/deficiency).

Even though these two different philosophies (Five Element and Eight Principles) lead to two very different diagnostic and treatment systems, they have a common foundational premise—parts can only be understood in relation to the whole. This is a stark contrast to western medical science that concerns itself with studies and experiments on specific biochemical relationships. The western medical focus is on correcting a specific biochemical aberration with a chemical medication and it matters little what the whole organism does or eats.

With the Eight Principles and the Five Elements it can be determined what diet, activity, climate, herb and other factors will alleviate or exacerbate a given condition. Oriental medicine and acupuncture will assist in promoting health and healing whatever the ailment.

Science or Art?

Oriental medicine fortunately contains both aspects—it is both science and art. There are certain aspects, such as using the tongue in oriental medicine diagnoses, that are more of a strict science. Other areas of oriental medicine, such as pulse diagnosis and the selection of which acupuncture points to use in treatment, are more of an art.

The best acupuncture point for any given condition is subject to the oddities and idiosyncrasies of an individual's spirit and energy system. The energy system of every individual is unique. Even though a person may have the same western disease label, the points and even the meridians used will be quite different. There are always several point combinations that will work well. Some will always be better than others and still others may be best.

The effectiveness of any treatment is dependent on three critical components: 1) The quality of energy inherent in the spirit that enlivens the body, 2) The practitioner's ability to assess what the person or spirit is asking for, and 3) The ability of the practitioner to provide the appropriate stimulus.

If the assessment is correct, there is still the task of choosing the points and techniques that will provide this intangible spirit quality. Acupuncture points are more than just numbers on a line. They all have their own personality and a name with a profound meaning. A point not only delivers a quantity of Qi, but has its own character and quality of energy. It takes a practitioner many years to get a sense of the personality for more than just a few points. The best acupuncturists take the scientific aspects of oriental medicine and enhance them in an artful way, blending science and objective information with wisdom and intuition or clairvoyance.

The basics aside, and with all training being equal, there are still vast differences in the way practitioners blend together art and science. If one practitioner's treatment didn't work, it doesn't mean that acupuncture doesn't work or that another acupuncturist can't help your particular problem. It just means, that particular treatment from that particular practitioner at that particular time didn't work for you. If you go to 50 different acupuncturists you are likely to receive 50 different treatments. They may or may not be similar treatments but they can all be beneficial. Undoubtedly some treatments will be more effective than others will.

It can't even be said that all acupuncturists use needles. Some practitioners may only use moxa or laser light. There is no one way to treat any one illness as each patient has a unique energy system. There is not any one technique in oriental medicine that needs to be used, as there are many ways to stimulate energy at the points and promote balance. Acupuncture points can be stimulated with needles, moxabustion, lasers, tuning forks, finger pressure, and other means. Different practitioners have affinities for different techniques. There are lots of different ways to get the job done, and it is up to the individual practitioner to use the techniques he or she feels suits the situation best.

It is very different than western medicine where one or two drugs are used to treat a particular diagnosis, and for good reason. No two illnesses are the same if you trace cause back to its true beginning.

Some acupuncturists are well trained while others, with just medical or dental degrees, have had only a few weekend workshops of acupuncture training. The state laws often allow medical professionals to use needles. These workshops are barely enough to learn point location but inadequate for learning diagnostic theory or treatment philosophy. Some states still do not have any regulation or licensure, but there is a national certifying agency—National Council for the Certification of Acupuncturists (NCCA). If the practitioner administering acupuncture is not certified by this organization, then chances are you didn't really receive an acupuncture treatment but rather were just stuck with needles.

The Five Element and Eight Principles philosophies represent two vastly different diagnostic and treatment systems within the acupuncture community. Most acupuncturists are trained in and practice one or the other. In order to find the best fit, the following information will be helpful.

Taoism, Yin, Yang, and the Five Elements

It is not the purpose of this book to go into depth about oriental medicine theory. There are other books listed in the bibliography that contain detailed information. The intention here is to give enough information so one can choose between different practitioners and styles of treatment, and know what questions to ask to achieve an appropriate fit.

There are many different diagnostic and treatment systems within the genre of oriental medicine. Here we will concern ourselves primarily with the systems of acupuncture. Ayurvedic medicine, which historically used acupuncture, does not include acupuncture in its scope today.

Acupuncture systems revolve around two major philosophies: Five Elements and Eight Principles. While they result in two very different styles of acupuncture, philosophically they do not contradict each other. They are really two aspects of the same philosophy—Taoism.

The Tao revolves around the notion that life is where Heaven and Earth intermingle. Tao is the means or the Way in maintaining harmony between this world and the beyond. The ancient Chinese believed that this harmony was crucial for good health. By shaping earthly conduct to correspond with the course of the universe, right living and good health would be achieved.

It was perceived that this universe was endowed with an all-powerful force and strength and was unforgiving toward ignorance and/or disobedience. At the very basis of this perception is the notion of duality or yin/yang, heaven/earth, sunny/cloudy, day/night, male/female and so on. The interaction of these dualistic elements is the basis and origin of movement and change.

Looking to nature to divine a course of right action, yin and yang were delineated into the Five Elements (metal, water, wood, fire, earth). The five elements become the basis for balance in defining the Tao. Each element is associated with a season as well as various qualities that are too numerous to mention here. A short list of elements and their associations are shown on the following page.

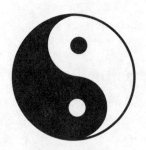

Table of Five Elements and Associations

	Metal	*Water*	*Wood*	*Fire*	*Earth*
Element					
Season	Fall	Winter	Spring	Summer	Late Summer
Direction	West	North	East	South	Center
Emotion	Grief	Fear	Anger	Joy	Sympathy
Sound	Weeping	Groaning	Shouting	Laughter	Singing
Color	White	Black/Blue	Green	Red	Yellow
Odor	Rotten	Putrid	Rancid	Scorched	Fragrant
Number	9	6	8	7	5
Planet	Venus	Mercury	Jupiter	Mars	Saturn
Organ	Lungs	Kidneys	Liver	Heart	Spleen
Climate	Dryness	Cold	Wind	Heat	Humidity

The character and quality of these associations provide guidance for right activity, the type of movement for particular seasons of the year. The wrong type of action at the wrong season would bring about an imbalance in the body's system and consequently discomfort or dis-ease. For example, winter is a yin season and is a time of coalescence and inactivity in order to renew our reserves. Consequently, if we undertake great activity in this period we won't have adequate resources in our body (an imbalance has been set up) for the great activity of spring and summer and we will have set the stage for injury.

The above table can also be used to guide treatment. If a patient has a lot of shout in their voice and an inability to experience joy and laughter, energy may need to be moved from the Wood channels to the Fire channels to restore balance.

The imbalances that result as a consequence of our activities are classified according to Eight Principles. These principles are Yin/Yang, Excess/Deficiency, Interior/Exterior, and Hot/Cold. An excess or deficiency in one of these elements not only creates a physical problem but results in an emotional imbalance that colors the entire personality of the individual. Emotional disturbances (depression or anxiety disorders) are usually early warning signs of a Qi imbalance.

For all practical purposes we are all born with an imbalance. Our energetic makeup at birth is determined by the energy we receive from our parents at conception, the spiritual energy we bring to this life and the cosmic energetic influences present at our particular time of birth. The qualities of these cosmic energetic influences can be ascertained by studying one's astrological influences.

Why would we start out in life with an imbalance? The degree of influence exerted upon our personality by particular elemental energies determines our personalities and consequently the type of experiences we will draw to us. These experiences provide us with learning and growth. We are provided with a rough direction for our life path or growth plan based on when and where we are born.

Five Element or Eight Principle

These two aspects of the Taoist philosophy over the years have given rise to two very different diagnostic and treatment systems. The **Five Element** system (also known as **Meridian Therapy**) focuses on color, sound, odor, and emotion. Pulses and symptoms are used to guide the practitioner in choosing which element is most in need of support. The emphasis is on tonification of the weak element. The **Eight Principles** approach focuses on the physical symptoms and the Eight Principles, paying particular attention to tongue diagnosis, with the pulses usually getting less attention than in the Five Element treatments. Eight principle style treatments usually address many elements and organ systems in one treatment with a greater emphasis on eliminating stagnation.

If you have had previous acupuncture treatments, the chances are it was an Eight Principle style treatment. Eight Principle style of acupuncture is the most commonly practiced form in this country as well as in China. Approximately 90 percent of acupuncturists use the Eight-Principle style of diagnosis and treatment. It is commonly known as **Traditional Chinese Medicine (TCM).** Although there are twenty or so acupuncture schools in the United States, only a few offer a full-blown Five-Element Program. The rest focus their core programs on TCM. There are postgraduate programs in Japanese style Five Element systems as well as elective courses and clinics at some of the TCM-based schools.

The major differences in treatment styles, as noticed by the patient, would be the radically different techniques of interviewing and needle insertion. The **Five-Element (5E)** interview will be more like a chat with a friend. In addition to symptoms, the practitioner will want to know about your relationships, your job, maybe where you like to go on vacation, or whatever you want to talk about. He or she will be looking more for out-of-place emotions, changes in color, voice inflection, and taking note of what you are asking for from a psychological/emotional point of view.

The **TCM** interview is more focused on physical signs, i.e., do you like cold or hot drinks, spicy or bland food, cold or hot rooms and so on. Is your urine clear or dark yellow, copious or scanty, and frequent or seldom? Are the menses regular, heavy, or no menses at all? Disturbed sleep? Do you have regular bowel movements, and are the stools soft and easy to pass or dry and difficult?

The tongue and pulses are also very important diagnostic indicators. The tongue is divided geographically into parts that correspond to the various organs. The color and coat of each area indicate the health and nature of imbalance in that organ. In oriental medicine there are twelve pulses, a yin and yang pulse for each element plus one for the Pericardium and Triple Burner channels. The practitioner assesses all the information, then puts the symptoms together to get a coherent picture of an energetic, organ/meridian imbalance. This imbalance is framed in the context of the person's overall constitution with the emphasis being on the weakest link, e.g., Lung deficiency, or a Kidney deficiency with Spleen deficiency being secondary.

These represent two different interview styles yet both arrive at an assessment of energetic imbalance of the human body/energy system from a holistic perspective. Both systems move energy to correct the imbalance. The TCM practitioner also uses herbs to correct the physiologic imbalance or to relieve symptoms. Unlike the western herbalist, the TCM formulas address the overall constitutional weakness and at the same time use herbs to treat the symptoms.

At this point the two systems may not seem significantly different. The real difference is felt while you are on the treatment table and after you get up from the treatment. In a TCM treatment, the needles are left in the body for 20 to 30 minutes, and sometimes longer. It is common to use 12 to 20 needles per treatment with some practitioners routinely using more than 30. The pulse is checked before the treatment. Some practitioners will check it again after the needles are removed, to assess what change has occurred and make any needed adjustments. Some TCM practitioners will not bother to check the pulse after the treatment. Some acupuncturists will not see the patient after the needles have been inserted. They have their assistants remove the needles. Others use electric stimulation, stick moxabustion, cupping and other techniques while the needles are in place.

There are at least three major different styles of 5E treatment systems: the European style as taught and developed by J. R. Worsley, the Japanese Meridian Therapy, and the Japanese Meridian Therapy as developed by the Toyohari Association. The most obvious differences are in the needling techniques. In a European style Five Element treatment the needles are inserted and removed within seconds or a soon as a Qi sensation is felt.

The Toyohari Association treatments are of particular interest because the needles are not inserted. Blind acupuncturists who had to do point location and needling technique by feel developed this non-insertion technique. As a result, they became very sensitive to energy and found better results working in the energy field just off the body.

The needle is held just above the acupuncture point or, in some instances, just touching the skin using a special technique. This technique actually results in better pulse changes and it is easier for the body to assimilate. Some patients miss the pain sensation of the needles but for most of us it is very enjoyable. The pulse is generally checked after each point is needled to verify the result. The quality of the pulse will determine if another point should be stimulated.

The pulse is again checked after the next point is treated and again when subsequent points are stimulated. It is like tuning up and adjusting a car that has twelve carburetors. The twelve pulses are very sensitive and reliable indicators as to how all officials (energetic/organ systems) of the body are running. When all systems are tuned, the treatment ends. The treatment could last 15 minutes or two hours.

There are some treatments where a 5E practitioner will leave needles inserted in the body but these are special instances that are needed relatively infrequently. Fewer points are selected. Often only two or three are needed to send a clear signal to the body to correct the imbalance. After the treatment the patient feels more organized and collected (clearer) than following a standard TCM treatment.

The 5E systems allow the practitioner to more finely tune the energy system and get better results. These techniques work particularly well in patients with emotional disorders, or basically healthy individuals who want to optimize their health and spiritual growth.

All systems promote energy movement to remove stagnation and work toward balancing the meridians and the body's energy system. Quite simply, the emphasis in TCM is on increasing circulation to tissues and organs with stagnant Qi. Tonification is used but is less directed because of the emphasis on circulation. Much of the tonification is achieved with herbs.

The Five-Element emphasis is on tonification in a very specific way that addresses the weak element with acupuncture. Energy stagnation is addressed by clearing Jaki with special techniques. Jaki is roughly translated as evil Ki (Qi) or aggressive energy. It is either cosmic debris that has penetrated to the meridian level or external energies that have been attracted by one's cosmic debris. Five Element practitioners rarely use herbs in their treatments.

Oriental Medicine in Summary

The origins of the two systems are lost somewhat in antiquity but at least some scholars report that acupuncture arose from the Five Element system. The Eight Principle system developed out of herbal treatment systems. In TCM, acupuncture points were later chosen to go with some herbal treatments based on the physical symptoms of the patient. Both systems are traditional and have the roots in ancient China and are based on ancient Chinese texts.

The only way for the uninitiated person to really know the difference is by the number of needles inserted. If many needles are inserted and left in place to circulate Qi in the body, then you received a TCM style treatment. If no needles are inserted but just touch the skin or are held over the point then you received a Japanese style Five Element treatment. If the needles were inserted but immediately and quickly withdrawn, then you received a European style Five Element treatment.

TCM style treatments have their best results with physical levels of illness such as musculoskeletal pain. It is a wonderful holistic model of medicine but lacks the fine tuning and qualities of the Five Element systems. Five Element, when done well, is pure poetry, the closest thing to a magic bullet this side of psychic healing. Five Element can operate on all levels: physical, mental/emotional and spiritual. Five Element is more effective for emotional problems and optimizing one's health. The refined Japanese style of Five Elements as taught by the Toyohari Association may be the best of all acupuncture treatments.

Ideally, a practitioner will be proficient in all three systems. This is still a rarity but it would be good if your practitioner is familiar with at least two of the three systems, and in some places we are quite lucky to have someone who is skilled in any of them. Most acupuncturists know a little of the other systems but usually focus on one or the other. The important question for the person seeking treatment is, what is the practitioner's specialty? What needling techniques are used? What is the basis of their training? Are they NCAA certified? Try different styles, if available, and see what resonates with you.

No matter what the illness, acupuncture and oriental medicine can be helpful.

A Word about Herbs

The body is a high performance organism and it deserves the best of foods and herbs. High quality fuel from food and herbs enables the body to perform optimally. However, with this said, herbs are rarely necessary. Few people have explored energetic healing options sufficiently so that they can say they **need** something more, to return to health.

Herbal medicines are similar to western drugs in that they are basically biochemical modifications. It brings to mind the story of the person who left the bath water running. The tub is overflowing and the water is filling the house. The panicked bather runs for the mop and is furiously mopping up the mess but forgets to turn the faucet off.

In illness the debris that is overloading and stressing the system and allowing the infection or other illness to flood the system remains unchanged. We begin mopping with drugs and herbals. It is quicker and easier, requires less thought and study or is cheaper than visiting the healer. In acute cases, one can mop and turn the faucet off as well. In the case of cancer one ought to be doing both or the body won't be around long enough to identify the issue that started the whole thing.

In many cases herbs are little more than special food. Many medicinal herbs are used in the kitchen. For healing purposes we often just need to alter the dose. There is a vast gray area between garlic in the kitchen and garlic in the treatment room. Then there is vast difference between garlic in the treatment room and tiger penis or rhinoceros horn in terms of global impact. Garlic is grown domestically and locally nearly anywhere in the world. The latter two products come from nearly extinct species. Many harvesters in any country value plants and animals solely for their market value. When we use herbs harvested from the wild anywhere, it is at great peril to the ecosystem and health of the planet. Since we have a connectedness to the ecosystem, depleting the plant life ultimately affects our own health.

For example, when we use the bark of a tree, we have no way of knowing if the bark alone or the entire tree was taken. Even if just the bark was removed, it may kill the tree. One would think they could just strip the bark from a limb without causing significant damage to the tree. However, many cases the entire tree is felled just to harvest the bark. Go figure! It must be efficient because many Chinese herbs are cheaper than toilet paper, but for how long.

So the decision to use herbs contains karmic implications as well. In many cases the illness is so severe and acute that herbs and/or drugs are necessary to give us the time to find the energetic solutions. To only seek out herbal remedies and ignore the underlying energetic/spiritual issues is folly on more than one level, especially if they are made from a rare and endangered species. As the wise old trapper once said—there is more than one way to skin a mule.

Speaking of mules, did you know that asshide glue, the scrapings from the under the skin of an ass, is an herb in the Chinese materia medica (E Jiao)? It used to nourish the blood, in treating dizziness and palpitations from deficient blood, and nourishes and moistens the lungs. It can stop many kinds of bleeding, especially consumptive bleeding of the lungs. At least mules are not an endangered species.

The Chinese have developed one of the most extensive materia medicas in the world, categorizing the tastes and functions for each herb including bat dung and earthworms, including what meridian they affect. Let's not forget centipedes, scorpions, cockroaches, geckos and other critters. The Chinese have analyzed and categorized practically everything you can put in your mouth as to how it will affect the human body. Will it make the body hotter or colder, more yin or yang, will it make Qi rise or sink, will it dry, moisten, or astringe? Which meridian will it enter and act upon, and to which organ will its healing properties be directed?

Every condition can be looked at in terms of these qualities. A herbal combination can be created to abate the symptoms as well as restore an overall balance to the body. Chinese herbs are rarely used singly; most herbal treatments are formulas consisting of from three to thirty herbs. The creating of formulas is as much of an art as it is a science, and each herbalist has his or her own favorite herbs.

Herbs are formulated to create the right balance for a given individual's constitution. Some herbs are added to offset the negative effects of other herbs. A good herbalist takes advantage of the synergism created from certain combinations. There is no one formula for the common cold that works for everybody. However, a basic formula can be adapted or altered to work best for a given individual's cold. For example, a person suffering from a common cold with a Lung Excess condition will need a different herbal formula than one with a cold and a Lung Deficiency. To someone not trained in TCM there wouldn't appear to be much of a difference. It's all about fine-tuning and using the right tool for the job.

In summary, illness and health operate as if it we are a cascade. Good health or ill health starts out like heaven above in our subtle energy layers and cascades downward through denser layers, finally reaching the physical layers of our being. Herbs operate on these denser layers, leaving the origins of disease untouched. In some acute situations we need to work on this layer with herbs or drugs at the same time we work on the subtle energetic layers.

Hydrotherapy (Bake Me)

Hydrotherapy is the natural way to move Qi. We're talking contrast hydrotherapy where you jump into the ice cold water after the hot tub, and then back into the hot tub, and back into the cold water, and back into the hot tub. Cycle through each at least three times (think laundromat), staying at least a minute in the cold and three minutes in the hot each time. It's a great way to generally circulate Qi and blood.

Many diseases start from stagnation. Hydrotherapy is just one of the many tools available to move Qi. Of course, exercise works great, too. Baking in a sauna and then taking a cold shower or a cold plunge in a pool has a similar effect, as long as core body temperature rises and falls at least a couple of degrees.

This is an example of affecting energetic change from the physical and cascading back to the energetic level. It starts with the circulation on the physical levels of blood and fluids, moves to the meridian level energies, and finally it has a slight impact on the more subtle levels. It will not balance your meridians or remedy any energetic deficiencies (cosmic or otherwise), but it does circulate your blood and Qi. This will not solve your spiritual dilemmas. It will help create a lighter energy so you can take a fresh look at them.

Colon Therapy (Plug Me into the Wall)

There are countless invasive procedures in medicine. Fortunately, I have experienced only a few them. In some peculiar way the sensation of being plugged into the wall is one I won't easily forget.

For those unfamiliar with this form of *therapy* you essentially plug a hose into your intestinal outlet, fill your intestines with water until you are about to burst, while the excess flushes back out. The fecal matter flows out into a machine that is connected to the waste pipes of the building's plumbing. The machine separates the waters entering and leaving you, preventing contamination from previous candidates. The machine is fitted with glass tubes so the attendant can monitor the quality of fecal matter as it passes. This is similar to an aquarium, especially if you have organisms living in your intestines. The feeling is one of intimacy with the facility's plumbing, a strange sensation to say the least.

The effect is to agitate your liver and gallbladder until they spill their contents. It's called a liver flush. The theory is that toxins from toxic chemical exposure accumulate in the liver. Flushing the liver releases the toxins. The intestine also benefits if it has accumulated years of heavy plaque buildup.

The downside of this treatment is that it devastates your Liver Qi, and takes a toll on the Qi of other organ systems as well, especially the Spleen. It takes weeks to rebuild your Qi after a colon therapy treatment. This is therapeutic for someone who has an intensely stagnated Liver with a body full of toxic chemicals. However, less invasive and drastic measures are easier for the body to assimilate.

Again, cleaning the energy in the subtle body enables the liver to release the toxins, especially when used in conjunction with dietary changes and herbal treatments. In working at a clinic where many very toxic patients underwent daily colonics for a month (with weekends off). While benefits were clear, there was also a cost. These patients had been exposed to silicone from leaking breast implants or poisoned with other toxic chemicals or herbs. In addition to colonics and acupuncture they received hydrotherapy, herbals, massage and other therapies.

Are severe treatments warranted for severely toxic bodies? In situations with physical level causes, physical level treatments are helpful. However, the energy system still acts on the physical body and can assist in the cleansing. Once again we are back with the muleskinner blues. Do you want to start at the head or just below the tail? The moral of this tale: petroleum products belong in machines like cars, silicone is great for caulking cracks, respect the dosages of herbs, and pesticides affect humans the same as pests.

Nineteen year-old female. Ingested Pennyroyal oil to induce abortion resulting in serious impairment of cognitive abilities, pronounced slowness of mental functioning. Many herbs do not have standardized quantities of active ingredient so it becomes difficult to accurately gauge the dose, especially when self-medicating without any training, as was the case with this woman. The above protocol of daily colonics, hydrotherapy, liver cleansing herbs, massage and acupuncture was carried out for one month. There was only slight improvement after the full course. The effects on the brain of using Pennyroyal may well be permanent.

Chapter 27

Working with the Woo Woo

I point to the moon, but you look at the pointing finger.
—Zen Koan

If we only knew who we are, I wouldn't be writing this book! We are spiritual beings with the ability to invite and be a conduit to the multitude of universal energies that exist. We can invite, focus, direct, send and channel an incredible array of vibrations at will. Some of these are healing, nurturing vibrations; others are incredibly destructive and toxic.

We actually invite energetic vibrations all the time whether we are conscious of it or not. One of the most common vibrations that we invite is competition. The competition vibration is encouraged in western society as if it is something positive and healthy. We couldn't be further from the truth. Competition was discussed previously in Chapter 13 at some length in *The Process of Becoming (Whacko)*. On the flip side, we can also invite compassion and love.

We invite or in some cases create these vibrations with our thoughts. We can invite these energies at will to assist us in our creations and to heal others and ourselves. Our ability to do this is limited only by our openness and state of mind. The more we do it, the more we understand the process, the more we trust it and the stronger it gets.

Healers from different cultures have used these healing energies for centuries in different ways yet it is fundamentally the same process. The process of channeling universal energies is really very simple. Mostly, you just need to lose your self-importance. The Chinese use medical Qi

Gong, the Japanese use Reiki, the Kahunas of Hawaii worked with channeled energy as well as other psychic techniques. No doubt many other healers unknowingly channel energy while they do massage or other bodywork.

Channeling energy is not to be confused with using your own healing energy to heal yourself. When we run our own energy for another's healing we become exhausted and, after a period of time, become ill ourselves. Many new practitioners eager to establish a clientele will unknowingly give up much of their own energy to heal their patients.

Natural Force Healing

Natural Force Healing is a system of working with channeled energies recently developed by Lisa and Dr. Kenneth Davis. Their techniques channel over 25 different vibrations of natural Positive Universal Flow Energies. A complete system of screenings and reflexes enables the practitioner to know the exact level or vibration needed, as well as to determine the issues creating the disease.

For example, a positive test in one of the screenings indicates that the individual is dealing with one of the following issues: inability to connect to their intuition, stuck in their heads, unable to be spontaneous, or to connect to the infinite. Further testing would narrow down which issue is actually causing the block. A particular energetic vibration would be channeled to open that aspect for the patient.

The objective of Natural Force Healing is more than keeping the body healthy or aiding the spirit in its journey. An important goal is to provide energetic lubrication for spiritual evolution so that we can smoothly slip over the sticky spots we encounter.

Lisa and Kenneth Davis have identified Five Fiery Elements of disease, which form a philosophical basis for their use of channeled energies for healing. These elements are summarized below:

1. Constriction

Constriction is caused by fear, making us unable to have faith and trust about the present and future, leaving us unable to share love and kindness for others.

2. Denial

Denial, particularly of the beauty of our higher essence and ourselves, becomes a deteriorating factor that leads to disease. Denial is one of those things nobody likes to admit taking part in. However, we all do it. The worst kind is denying that we even have a higher spiritual self. Unfortunately, our society has taught us that we are just of body and mind, showing little concern of how to nurture the spiritual body.

Nurturing the spiritual could allow us the conscious ability to transcend with the physical into the spiritual realms of reality. Many times, as children in such a structured society, we lose our ability to be individuals and free thinkers so as not to lose pace with our peers. Hence we evolve late or not at all in many areas of our self-awareness. We often deny our true feelings in order to please, impress others, or in fear of rejection or reprisal. Our lives are based on the moment; we cannot live in or change the past or future. Much of our lives are wasted in either of these two realms of consciousness.

3. Evolution of the Soul

We manifest in a physical and spiritual form for a purpose. The physical body is the vehicle that allows the spirit to transform and manifest its reality for our evolution. It is important to realize the reformation of the spirit is a conscious decision. Refraining from doing conscious wrong and doing good only for our own well-being is the fight of our whole existence. We must awaken to understand the impact of our choices.

4. Abstaining From Life

We were created to participate in this challenge called life. Most of us are so wounded that we want to retreat someplace safe, withdrawing into our own little world. Each and every person matters as an individual and is part of the whole. We are all interconnected in more ways than you could imagine. Without participation in life, we lose our will and ability to thrive. When we don't thrive, we die a little bit each day, causing our own subconscious doom and breakdown. Sharing and openly receiving inspiration ignites change.

5. Abusive Nature

Through all of it we have survived! People are not only abusive to themselves, but to all of their kind in trying to find fault instead of similarities, overwhelming all of our senses to the point of destruction and encouraging others to follow suit. Tragically, we are taught to be abusive by our times and society. It's actually socially acceptable! Many comedians and journalists command great respect and high fees for their prowess at being abusive. Most don't even have an inkling of their own abusiveness. We are taught to work hard and play even harder, in order to belong and to acquire. As a result we have lost our sense of peace, simplicity and the deep need for spiritual tranquillity.

Natural Force Healing in Summary

The connection between the philosophy of Natural Force Healing and why a certain individual needs a particular level is not immediately obvious to the practitioner. Understanding the connection between each vibration and its relationship to the Five Fiery Elements involves some complicated study. However, every nuance need not be fathomed for a practitioner to use the system successfully. A practitioner merely uses muscle testing to screen for the appropriate treatment levels for an individual. Determining the levels also informs the practitioner about the patient's current growth period.

For example, the description for one level or vibration used in treatment is "Spiritual Adherence Technique—will allow an individual to adhere to spiritual laws as well as coming to know God." This vibration would make it difficult for the patient to continue with abusive behavior, and have other benefits as well.

Another level is called "Omnipresence—displays the depth of our spiritual awakening." It allows us the ability to be reunited within the essence and memory of new life. In other words, these energies provide you with the energetic material that you need to continue on with your spiritual evolution or transformation.

Positive Universal Force Energies provide important building blocks for physical health and well-being. Most importantly they provide not just any random energetic vibration but the most limiting factors in your physical and energetic bodies.

Chapter 28

I have given each being a separate and unique way of seeing and knowing and saying that knowledge.
—Rumi recounting Gods revelation to Moses

Psychic Healing

Since the word psychic has many ethereal connotations it may help to pin down just what we are talking about. According to Webster's dictionary the word *psychic* comes from the Greek word *psychikos* meaning spiritual, or of the soul. This in turn comes from the Greek *psyche* (breath, life, or soul) which derived from *psychien* to breathe, blow. The word psychic is defined then as that which pertains to the psyche, or soul, lying outside the realm of physical forces.

Webster's dictionary also defines *soul* as the actuating or animating principle of the individual life. This has striking similarity in meaning to the Chinese word Qi, the Japanese Ki, the Sanskrit Prana that all translate as life force, breath of life, enervating life principle and so on. In oriental medicine, Qi is understood in terms of its function within diagnosis and treatment of real patients with real problems. Little attention is given to theoretical description or modeling outside of this context. The ideas of the role Qi plays in acupuncture are pragmatically tested and examined for validity and consistency. Functionally, it is seen as an enlivening principle.

In his book, *Religiousness and Yoga*, T.K.V. Desikachar defines Prana as "that which is constantly present everywhere." Furthermore he states "Prana has an intimate relationship with the mind" thus "Prana, mind and breath are interrelated. Whatever happens in the mind influences the breath." The Yoga Sutra uses the word Purusa as many in the west use the word spirit. *Purusa* may be thought of as that which understands. Not that which knows, not the memory function of the brain, but that which understands. Again Desikachar says, "Prana is simply the expression of Purusa in all parts of the body and beyond." In expression there is information.

A psychic person, according to Webster's dictionary, is someone who is sensitive to nonphysical or nonmaterial forces. Putting this all together we see the psychic as someone sensitive to the information expressed in Qi or Prana. Many acupuncturists, when they read the pulses, are reading beyond the physical sensation of the pulse. They are actually reading the information present in the Qi without consciously intending to do so. When clairvoyants do a reading, they are actually reading the information present in these Qi or Pranic fields.

Psychic healing does not use material forces, i.e., needles, herbs, physical manipulation, homeopathics or drugs. For the purpose of simplicity, channeled energies are not included in this section. Channeled energy therapies such as Healing Touch, Reiki, or Natural Force Healing certainly involve working with nonmaterial energies but they do not require sensitivity to the information contained within these fields. Even though this information may be used for assessment, through energy-sensing scopes or muscle testing, it does not involve the translation of the information within the individual's sixth chakra.

Psychic healing is an incredibly vast reservoir of untapped potential in the field of medicine and healing. The nonphysical is virtually where all illness begins. Yes, even genetic disorders—your genetic makeup is simply your spiritual energetic history mixing with that of your parents' spiritual energetic history and manifesting as biochemistry.

As mentioned earlier, your aura and chakras contain vast amounts of information about you and your activities—past, present, and future. A clairvoyant or psychic is simply someone who naturally or through training understands how to access and interpret this reservoir of information. It is stored in subtle energy patterns similar to the latest holographic storage devices in computers. It is probably only a matter of time before instruments connected to computers can read what is stored in your aura. If the reservoir of stored information is pure and clean, we are unlikely to experience health problems.

This reservoir is not just a pile of dead information. It is the body's operating system just like the operating system in the computers we use.

If the operating system has bugs in it as computer operating systems do, we begin producing cosmic debris that pollutes the reservoir of information. This debris creates illness. Clearing the debris and debugging the operating system is the work of Psychic Healing.

Studying the color of the aura will tell us what "stuff" is in the reservoir of the aura. Analyzing the color of the aura is similar to analyzing the exhaust or smoke emitted by a car's engine. The information within the aura is much more detailed than whether an engine is running rich or lean. Everything that you have ever done or thought is recorded in your energy system. This all has an impact on how cleanly, smoothly and powerfully your body performs.

Each cylinder (chakra) puts out its own smoke in a distinct layer. The range of colors is the full spectrum. Each color posesses a different vibration and each vibration represents a different issue. A clairvoyant reader will also receive symbols and/or pictures that depict the flavor of the day—the issue that person is working with at that particular point in time. This is a simplified version of what a *reader* or psychic healer does. There are many other aspects to a reading and how this information aides healing, but readings are best experienced rather than intellectualized.

All fine and good, where does the healing come in? Actually, it already happened and you didn't even know it. Without going any further with psychic healing techniques, the energy system of the body was changed from the reading. A reading in and of itself is often enough to begin clearing the debris. A clairvoyant reading communicates information directly to spirit. The action of being seen clairvoyantly profoundly impacts our energetic body in a healing way.

In addition, revealing yourself as spirit with all your baggage and not being judged is very healing. What is it that we are all looking for so desperately? Is it not to be seen and accepted or loved? Many people go through their whole lives without being looked at for anything other than the clothes they wear, how their hair is done, their career, what possessions they own and so forth. A clairvoyant reading provides an opportunity to be seen without judgement and for many of us that is healing in itself.

Readings also move stagnant energy. Energy movement is healing because it relieves the stress that stagnation creates on the physical level.

Some types of energetic movements are more healing than others are. It depends on the particular level of the stagnant energy. If the stagnation is on the meridian level, then an acupuncture treatment will be more effective than an aura combing or reading and vice versa. In general, the rule is that movement is healthier than stagnation.

Mental activity is not the movement discussed here. The brain, occupied with thinking, does move energy. But in a different context. Mental activity is usually an escape from dealing with the issue (the stagnation) at hand, and only creates more stagnation in the energy system.

Think of a frozen river in springtime. As the river thaws, large chunks of ice flow downstream catching on logs and forming a jam. Most of the thinking we do, unless it is meditative inquiry, is like bringing in a bulldozer and adding more snow and ice to the dam. In many cases, we add a few logs and boulders and then pack it down good and hard.

That first log in the stream is analogous to that first childhood wound. We all have had many wounds and so there are many logs in the river for the ice flows to get hung up on. Readings move energy at the deeper levels of our soul or spirit, and this is healing.

A reading brings up the energy and issue held in that ice jam, clearing the hang ups and absurdities through insight and understanding. Once we understand the issue hanging up our ability to love, it sets the jam free. This is change. This is healing. The energy is free to flow again. This can be very dramatic, with lots of tears, and emotions or even shaking.

Streaming—Shake Rattle and Roll

Shaking is a process that tends to scare people, especially those with western medical training. When deep energetic blocks are set free, the energy rushes through the body with great force, stimulating nerve centers and making the limbs move in a spastic fashion. Some practitioners call this streaming.

Streaming is generally a healthy response and not to be confused with Parkinson's Disease, epileptic seizures or the tremors that are associated with Liver Wind (Liver Wind is a condition in oriental medicine that results from Liver Qi congestion) or liver disease. These shaking episodes can last a few seconds or several hours.

The Shakers built a religion around this phenomenon. It can happen once in a lifetime or every day for years. It can be triggered by a religious experience, during bodywork, acupuncture, rebirthing or practically any healing modality. Shaking can start suddenly on its own or seemingly out of the blue. It depends on the nature of the block, who you are and how much energy is behind the jam.

Sedating the body with drugs stifles and stops the healing process. Adding a tranquilizer or anticonvulsant to the system is like dumping a bucket of sludge, bumble gum, and hair into a toilet. The flush just isn't going to happen. You will only create more of what the body is trying to clear from its system.

The western disease known as epilepsy has a similar etiology but differs from the spasms or tremors associated with a healing release. Epileptic seizures usually create a greater rigidity, often a loss of consciousness, and disorientation after the seizure. Epileptics frequently suffer from the so-called bipolar disorder, chaarcterized by periods of mania with great emotional strength or cockiness followed by periods of timidity and weakness.

To the clairvoyant, these episodes of emotional swings correspond with an opening and closing of the third chakra. The third chakra is about honor and integrity. The third chakra is also the main energy distribution center of the body so when it closes it creates a serious backup of Qi. Clinical experience has shown that most people experience only partial restrictions in the third chakra.

In the epileptic, the third chakra closes down almost entirely resulting in feelings of great timidity. When this happens the body can't function, and the amount of energy backing up is just too strong for the restriction. The chakra is forced open, resulting in feelings of great power or even mania. If the backup and release are very severe the chakra "blows a gasket" and the release becomes quite violent with enough spiritual energy leaving the body so as to produce a loss of consciousness.

This event is so traumatic that spirit leaves the body, taking consciousness with it. The epileptic completely disoriented after a seizure needs time for spirit to return to the body. The challenge for healing is to help the epileptic recognize what aspect of his belief system shuts him down. This enables the epileptic to regulate his energetic swings himself.

Blue Envelope

The Blue Envelope is a denser layer of energy just off the surface of the body (acupuncturists call it Wei Qi). It is part of the etheric body also called the etheric template or the etheric double. The Blue Envelope keeps the energy system intact and coherent. It protects us from foreign energies.

If your Blue Envelope has holes in it, you will be sensitive to all kinds of toxins in the environment. These toxic assaults come from many sources such as electronic smog, chemical pollution, and the harmful thoughts of others. These holes can be created by anger, our own lewd thoughts, abusive behavior, others harmful thoughts and harsh judgments, radiation of various kinds, and the sudden release of strong, pent-up emotions.

Environmentally sensitive individuals usually have many holes in their blue envelope. A clairvoyant can look at a person's blue envelope and can see the holes and then psychically patch them. There are also techniques within the Natural Force Healing System to repair holes in the Blue Envelope. Even though the various systems of acupuncture recognize this layer of energy, the acupuncture techniques are less effective at diagnosing the extent and nature of damage as well as treating the underlying problem.

Astral Body

The astral body is the energetic aspect of yourself leaves the physical body while you sleep. Much of our dream world is actually our adventures on the astral plane, a level of existence where we can create instantaneously. When we are out of our bodies, we encounter other energetic phenomena that can damage our astral body. The damage or toxic energy can be transferred to our physical bodies upon our return.

Have you ever awoken feeling as if you had been run over by a truck? Well, maybe you were. Those stiff necks that we associate with sleeping "wrong" may be injuries from the astral layer. Again, this toxic debris can be cleansed with psychic healing techniques. These techniques do not translate to print very well, they really need to be communicated experientially in a classroom setting.

53-year-old male presenting with hemorrhoids, boils, poor digestion, spontaneous sweating, many food allergies, candidiasis, muscle spasm and tightness around rectum, history of hepatitis. Deficient Lung and Spleen pulses with an excess Liver pulse. Treatment with acupuncture and Chinese herbs was focused on tonifying the digestive system while detoxifying and decongesting the liver. Treatments were once every two weeks for six months then once a month for a year.

After the first year of treatment most symptoms cleared, especially boils, hemorrhoids, digestion, and food allergies. The tight muscles in the rectal area persisted in spite of vigorous acupuncture and deep tissue work. The patient at this point was scheduled for surgery in two days, to cut the muscles in the rectal area to relieve the spasm.

At this point I was becoming more adventurous with psychic healing and decided to "take a look" as we say. There was much inflammation on the astral body in the area of the rectum. This energy was cleared psychically. The muscle spasm and inflammation of the colon subsided almost immediately. When the surgeon inspected the previously inflamed rectum two days later, the inflamation was 95 percent reduced. There was no need for surgery. It is one of those miracle cures where all you see is this person waving his hand in the air and a cure has happened. If you understand the energy system of the body, it's no miracle at all.

Chapter 29

Your loving doesn't know its majesty,
Until it knows its helplessness.
— Jelaluddin Rumi

Healing with Color and Crystals

The *New Age* brings revived attention to color therapy, aromatherapy, homeopathy and similar healing techniques. The origins of color therapy can be traced back several hundred years to Ayurvedic medicine. Ayurvedic medicine treatments incorporated the use of different colored gemstones. Each gem has a unique color and vibration. The gem's crystalline structure and physical shape focuses and amplifies its energy. A crystal with a broken tip would serve to diffuse energy instead of focusing it.

Gems are one of many color-based energetic healing tools. Colors are specific vibrations of energy, similar to those of an earthquake. Earthquakes vary in intensity. Some earthquake vibrations are more effective at breaking up buildings than others are. For example, some vibrations are more effective at breaking up brick buildings while others are more effective at destroying earth or wood frame structures. Different colors, with different vibrations, will break up different kinds of energetic blockages in the body.

Different emotional and health issues create different blockages. These blockages revolve around belief systems or thought conglomerates. Belief systems are not truth and actually exclude truth and understanding. Each has its own energetic structure and vibration, therefore requiring different vibrations to clear them. This blockage, as the name implies, creates stagnation in the energy system with toxic buildup at the cellular level.

When there are no blockages and our energy is flowing freely, blood, fluid and nutrients flow freely in and out of the tissues and cells. Different colors will activate or stimulate different aspects of cellular metabolism. Microorganisms such as viruses and bacteria have vibrations in which they thrive. Other vibrations inhibit their growth.

Some vibrations will promote health more than others. The effectiveness of the color being used will depend on what each person's tissues need at that time. Higher and lighter energies are generally more effective at promoting movement and health than are dark heavy vibrations (i.e. murky dark green). However, if you have a murky dark green in your aura, since like vibrations attract like vibrations, running a dark green will help pull out the dark green that is already present.

There are at least two different ways of working with color, internally or spiritually generated color and externally generated color such as colored light bulbs, colored water, and colored walls. Spiritually generated cosmic energy of whatever color you specify is the most efficient and cost effective way to produce great results. It certainly is environmentally friendly and the most affordable health care in the cosmos. Free for all, once you know how. There are some applications where externally generated color may be more effective, such as when working with eyesight.

Employing gemstones is one way to tap a source of external energy. However, it is actually the same cosmic energy that we can generate spiritually using psychic techniques. The type and color of the crystal externally determine the vibration. Healers working without stones, instead using psychic techniques, can identify and channel the energy the patient needs. Crystals and stones can be charged or programmed with various vibrations both intentionally and unintentionally.

Crystals readily pick up the energies of the surrounding environment. These foreign energies then mask the original vibration of the stone. If the stone has been in a room of angry people it will pick up some of that angry vibration. Therefore, a crystal used for healing should be cleansed after each use. Leaving it in the sun or in salt doesn't really do the job. Proper cleansings require psychic techniques to remove unwanted debris.

If a crystal can create a vibration, then we can also create it as spirit without the crystal. Any healing that can be done with a crystal can also be done more simply and nearly as powerful using other techniques. The use of crystals is not necessary, and more often than not is harmful. We don't have much control over the quality of energy coming through a crystal. Often we are contaminating the healing energy by exposure to debris held within the crystal.

Stones do not have to be crystals to hold a charge and affect our energy. A common river stone can be handled to fix a charge within it. There are ways to make this charge permanent. If a woman handles it then it will have a different vibration that if a man handles it. Putting three charged stones in a line creates an energy field between them, which will store various energetic vibrations that pass through it for ill or benefit.

In Scotland there are many cairns of charged rocks built in a straight line for great distances across the countryside. There is a measurable line of energy present between these cairns, which is known as a *ley line*. J. Havelock Fidler in his book, *Earth Energy*, has researched this phenomenon at considerable length. Fidler also discovered that seeds sprouted more slowly over these energy lines. The ensuing plant would then grow up to be a stunted specimen as well. However, if the charged stone was magnetic then a synergistic effect occurred enabling the plants to sprout and grow faster than normal.

In summary, gems, crystals, and even stones affect subtle energies that in turn affect our bodies for positive or negative results. The whole business is largely a cumbersome and unnecessary affair. Spiritual techniques yield results with less fuss and greater control. The case of Diamond Lil below illustrates the kind of damage that can occur with gems.

> *Sixty three year-old female, complaining of sciatica pain (pain running from low back through the buttocks and down the back or outside of the leg). Lil also had a host of other problems from fatigue, depression, fibromialgia and the like. Lil walked very stiffly, half bent over, with a gray, lusterless complexion. The most noticeable feature was the four diamond rings she wore on her hands. These were not your ordinary diamond rings, these were big ones. The smallest was*

about six carats and the largest about ten. A ten-carat diamond is about the size of a dime.

Up until this time I never thought much about the stones people wore, I just assumed the effect they had on people was rather negligible. I had read Fidler's book and taken a workshop but had no real first hand experience.

When Lil walked in, much to my dismay the first words out of my mouth were, "Are those diamonds? Are they real?" She replied, "Oh yes, this one, the rectangular one I bought from a famous hollywood producer, this one I bought from a prostitute who robbed many of her clients so she could buy it." There were many more in the collection that she kept in a safe deposit box. Each stone had its own story.

She was a fun unpretentious person, dressed very inexpensively. Well, I was impressed. I had never seen one stone that size let alone four on one hand. I thought that was the end of it.

I proceeded with the interview. She had so many symptoms that I decided to first take a look clairvoyantly and clean off her astral body. When I closed my eyes to read the only things I could see were the diamonds. Bright, shiny diamonds everywhere. Regardless of what was at the root of her problems, the diamonds had to be dealt with first. I had her remove them and looked again. Her astral body looked like Swiss cheese—nothing but holes. When I asked for a picture of what this was about I saw the diamonds again.

I began to psychically clean the diamonds. The room lightened up as the filthy toxic energy from many different people started to clear. The pain from previous owners had accumulated in the diamonds over the years. The one from the prostitute even had a curse on it. Curses require a little extra work to clear and this one came with many sordid pictures. Repairing the astral body, clearing the diamonds and charging them with healing vibrations, in addition to acupuncture, was the first treatment. She felt much better the next week, with more energy and emotionally in better place. However, the sciatica pain still persisted.

Three more acupuncture treatments relieved some of the sciatic pain. If the problem was simply an energetic disturbance with physical trauma, the sciatica would have been gone by now. It was not. It was time to look deeper once again. The clairvoyant picture was of a man riding in a diaper fashioned like a swing. It was attached at the hips by a spike. Ouch, big spikes too. Spikes that would give anybody sciatic pain.

The guy in the diaper, it turned out, was her investment broker. She thought he'd been ripping her off for years. It certainly looked like he was getting a free ride from where I sat. I cleared the energy and the sciatic pain was better. After six treatments she was greatly improved, with more energy, a happier disposition, and luster returning to her complexion. The sciatic pain was nearly gone. Obviously the problem will not clear completely until she finds another broker or deals with him differently.

We shouldn't expect too much, too soon from our patients. They all heal in their own time. After six visits she told her church about these treatments. The good God-fearing folks that they were made her stop coming. Psychics and the like are the work of the devil or some such thing. Thou shall not read thy Qi! Amen.

Chapter 30

The real voyage of discovery consists not in seeking new lands but in seeing with new eyes.

—Marcel Proust

Reconnection

The concept of maintaining healthy energy is very simple, just be *simple*. When you inherit a consciousness that is steeped in *becoming*, instead of being simple, it is the hardest work there is. The ego just won't have it. Our ego demands that we become at least respectable if not great, whatever that might mean to the individual. We create great convoluted schemes and structures around *becoming* secure or *being somebody*. Somebody of importance, prestige and notoriety because we think this will make everything turn out good, or "fun." In a word "secure." This process of becoming removes us from present time and attracts all sorts of unhealthy and ungodly debris. It confounds and confuses the mind, which in turn fills the body with a mess of out of time energy.

To heal is to step out of that time bound consciousness and connect to "what is". Energetically that means connecting to the source or the ground from which we originally came. Practically it means giving voice and expression to our passions (not emotions) even if they are a bit embarrassing. This doesn't mean we act out every abusive or violent thought, but we let them surface and explore their origins and motivation.

Intellectually it means abandoning all belief and organized religion including its ethics. Instead you simply are religion, you embody religiousness. It doesn't matter what that looks like, whether you call it God, Jehovah, Allah, or Phhhth. Better not to call it a name at all, just be with the energy.

171

Health is directly related to the reality of making that energetic connection. Finding the source of pure clean energy that is uncontaminated by time and thought. It is not some far off state attainable only by the few enlightened ones. That state of " " is all around us, hidden only by the process of becoming.

We may call it love, we may call it forgiveness or compassion. It matters not what we call it for it is not the word. It is the clarity of vibration, the clarity of what is seen that matters. Without this essence, life is a trip, an experience, a journey, or a smorgasbord of different energies to invite into your space. One may find great pleasure in sampling the flavor of each but in the end there is only one energetic vibration, one state that will truly satisfy our hunger. When that vibration is in us, we are that. We are individuals in many superficial ways but at the core we all drink from the same well.

Reconnecting with our source brings fresh clean energy just as the clouds fill the reservoir with fresh water. It is as this point that our potential for creating beauty can begin to develop. Is the drive in living matter to perfect itself really a drive to discover what beauty we can create? Are there limits to beauty? Is there an absolute beauty? Yes, there is a perverse kind of beauty in the chaos that engulfs the planet at present. It teaches us a great deal about the nature of consciousness. At least some aspects of it show us who we are in the context of stress and violence. There is another aspect of consciousness that has been largely unexplored so far in earth history, the aspect of cooperation and thinking together. With reconnection this arena becomes the new frontier and the beauty that will be born will be greater than anything yet seen on earth.

Glossary

ACTUALITY – That which exists in nature with or without your thoughts and emotional influence. The aspects of the cosmos that exist without you or your personal spin. Your existence is, however, part of that existence. Objective reality.

ARROGANCE – The state that arises with belief. The condition necessary for the birth of fear.

AURA – Kinesthetic medium or energy field generated by the chakras surrounds the body. It contains vast amounts of information.

BECOMING – The psychological process of imitating the ideal in order to become secure. In truth, it is only a stick and carrot routine. You can only be what you are. It is a futile exercise in chaos. This is not to be confused with practicing golf or tennis to be the best the world has ever seen.

BLUE ENVELOPE – The layer of subtle energy just off the body by about an inch. It surrounds and protects the body and energy system from invasion. In Oriental medicine it is called Wei Qi which translates as Defensive Qi.

CLAIRVOYANCE – Clear seeing. The process of using your sixth chakra to access information from other dimensions. Gives one the ability to tell Truth from a Lie. The power of discerning objects that are not present to the senses but have objective reality or actuality. Perspicacious.

CLAIRVOYANT – One who translates subtle energy into visual and then verbal information.

EVIL QI – Bioenergy that possesses qualities that are injurious to the body.

GROUND – Energy systems need a ground in order to complete a circuit. Since energy is neither created nor destroyed we need a ground so we have a place to send unwanted energies. We can ground either to the earth or up to spirit. It also provides us with a sense of connectedness to the earth or to spirit. It is very stabilizing for the body.

LIE – Utterances known to be false. The concept that forms the basis for any belief whether conscious or not. Assumption.

NATURE – That which is not put together with thought. Also Natural.

NINE STEPS TO BECOMING – The psychological movement of violence broken down into nine steps. The consciousness that we all share.

OFFICIAL – The personality associated with each organ system. (i.e., the Emperor is associated with the heart, the ruler of all in the kingdom, makes sure everyone is taken care of before himself).

OPINION – Fictitious statements that are believed to be true by the idiots espousing them. An intellectual construct. Forgive the bluntness, but the American notion that "everybody is entitled to their own opinion" is sheer idiocy. A greater falsehood has never been told and accepted with such ubiquity. Espousing a statement that may or may not be true, as if were fact, can only lead to conflict and war. If we had the good sense to explore and inquire as to the nature of the concepts that occur to us then the dynamic of relationship would have a whole new look.

PAIN PICTURE – A memory of past invalidation carried forward to present time for the purpose of creating perfect pictures. The basis for aversion behavior, the birth of the process of becoming.

PERFECT PICTURE – The ideal, the basis for desire.

PSYCHIC – One who can translate the information held in subtle energy fields into pictures that point to phenomena.

QI – A symbol depicting the vibratory continuum of matter and energy. This continuum behaves as if of ethereal waves and energetic nature. That vital force that enlivens and/or embodies.

REALITY – That which makes up your own personal experience, including your thought/emotions. All aspects of being that influence your world whether or not they exist outside of your imaging faculties or not.

SELF – Thoughtform conglomerate that depicts a concept of who we are.

SILVER CORD – Energetic tether between spirit and body. Designates ownership of a particular body by a particular spirit.

SPIRIT – A quasi-energetic entitiy that exists within and/or without a body. Spirit has consciousness with or without being attached to a body.

SPACE – AKA OUR SPACE – Our space includes our physical body, our aura, and our ground.

SPIRITUAL INFORMATION – Information available to us as spirit from other dimensions ("the other side") and other realities as well as this one. This includes our past lives as well as those of others; this information is then made intelligible to our human mind through interpretation in the sixth chakra usually in the form of a picture. One can also receive spiritual information audibly through the fifth chakra.

THOUGHT FORM CONGLOMERATE – Bundle of energy and/or information that is composed of thoughts and elementals.

TRUTH – That which cannot be denied. That which is not of an intellectual nature, not put together by thought. Cannot be proven by science only seen in moments of revelation by those who are good enough to look. How can you tell the difference between someone coming from the truth and someone who is espousing an opinion? See clairvoyant.

Further Reading

Braving the Void: Journeys into Healing. Dr. Michael Greenwood. Victoria, B.C.: PARADOX, 1997 (1980 Cromwell Rd. Victoria B.C. BC V8P 1R5)

The Dream Book: Symbols for Self-Understanding. Betty Bethards. Rockport, MA: Element, 1995.

Eagles of the New Dawn. Patricia Pereira. Hillsboro, OR: Beyond Words, 1997.

Ida Rolf Talks. Edited by Rosemary Feitis. Boulder, CO: Rolf Institute, 1978.

The Impossible Question. J. Krishnamurti, New York, NY: Harper and Row, 1972.

Natural Force Healing. Transformation of Consciousnes for our Evolution. Lisa V. Davis and Dr. Kenneth Davis.

PEACE PILGRIM: Her Life in Her Own Words. Compiled by Friends of Peace Pilgrim. Hemet, CA: Friends of Peace Pilgrim, 1994.

The Psychic Healing Book. Amy Wallace and Bill Henkin. Oakland, CA: Wingbow Press, 1996.

Religiousness in Yoga T.K.V. Desikachar. Lanham, MD: University Press of America, 1980.

Sex and Psychic Energy. Betty Bethards. Petaluma, CA: Inner Light Foundation, 1977.

Understanding Acupuncture. Stephen J. Birch, Robert L. Felt, Churchill Livingstone, 1999.

The Web That Has No Weaver. Ted J. Kaptchuk, New York, NY: Congdon and Weed 1983.

You Can Heal Your Life. Louise L. Hay. London, England: Eden Grove Editions, 1988.

The Zen Taching of Huang Po. Translated by John Blofeld. New York, NY: Grove Press, 1958.

About Ibis Healing Arts

Ibis Healing Arts School of Spiritual and Energetic Healing is located in Colorado Springs, Colorado. Our goal is to provide the modern healer with training and understanding in state of the art energetic healing techniqes and philosophies.

The clinic offers treatment through various modalities including acupuncture, oriental medicine massage, Core Integration, Natural Force Healing, cranial sacral therapy, Qi gong shiatsu, yoga instruction, self-healing classes, psychic healing, and clairvoyant readings.

The school currently offers coursework in self-healing philosophy and experiential techniques, core integration therapy, medical Qi gong, psychic healing, yoga, and clairvoyant training. Future course offerings will include acupuncture, massage, astrology, and herbology.

To contact Randall Leofsky at Ibis Healing Arts for appointments, classes, or to schedule a workshop:

Ibis Healing Arts
719-329-1618
www.healforreal.com

Index